CONTENTS

I would like to thank my husband, Chad, and the rest of my family, Jim, Sherry, Dan, and Dani, for their continued love, support, and motivation to write this book.

PREFACE

I have been competing in triathlons and marathons for fourteen years and have yet to find a comprehensive nutrition guide for triathletes. I am continually amazed at how much time triathletes spend making sure they have the right gear, optimizing their training plans, or selecting races that have courses designed to help them achieve a personal record (PR). Yet, the one thing I see most triathletes overlook or ignore completely is their nutrition.

Nutrition can be overwhelming to the average athlete. There is so much information and advice out there—much of it not very good—that it's sometimes difficult to sift through all of it and make the right nutrition choices. Some athletes also simply think that what they put into their bodies doesn't have much impact on their physical performance.

I wanted to teach others the nutrition secrets and information I learned as a triathlete, so I decided to combine my knowledge in nutrition and exercise physiology with my race experience to write this nutrition guide for my fellow triathletes. It doesn't matter whether you are a first-time participant or an experienced triathlete, whether you are training for a Sprint distance or an Ironman—this book will help ensure that you cross that finish line with the best nutrition plan possible. The knowledge you gain from this book should be practiced and implemented as an important component of your training plan and race-day performance. So, happy training—and remember that you can only be as good as your nutrition allows!

INTRODUCTION

Have you ever started the run portion of a triathlon and wondered where you were going to find the energy to finish? Or, have you ever hit the wall during a race and wondered if you'd even be able to finish at all?

Let me introduce two runners to you: Runner one is an eighteen-year-old female competing in her first marathon. She runs a fairly flat race course in temperatures of 70 to 80 degrees Fahrenheit. Her final race time is 4 hours, 37 minutes. Runner two is a twenty-year-old female competing in her second marathon. She runs a fairly flat race course in temperatures of 50 to 60 degrees F. Her final race time is 3 hours, 50 minutes. At first glance, you might conclude that runner two is probably a better, faster runner; however, while runner two does have the experience of one marathon under her belt, that experience wouldn't account for the entire forty-seven minutes shaved off of her time.

Now, what if I told you that runner one and runner two were actually just one person—me? That's right; runner one was me, after my first marathon; runner two was me after my second, a whole forty-seven minutes faster than my first one. Anyone who has completed a marathon will recognize that this is a huge improvement. So, what was the difference? Simple: my race nutrition.

I did my first marathon when I was eighteen, fresh out of high school, with no knowledge whatsoever about fueling during endurance exercise. The only thing I did know was that you weren't supposed to try anything new on race day that you hadn't done in practice. I had never consumed anything other than water during my training runs, so that's all I had on race day. Unfortunately, my tank ran out of gas at about mile 21, and I walked / painfully jogged the last 5 miles. To date, I think those 5 miles were the longest of my life. It was a good lesson, though. I saw runners all around me (and flying by me) who ate and drank calories quite regularly. I figured they must be on to something. I did my research after that, and although I still didn't fuel properly for my second marathon, my race nutrition was much better. The results spoke for themselves.

In the years since, I have cut another thirty minutes off that second marathon time, and I've been competitive in the sport of triathlon, with races ranging from Sprint to Ironman distances. I attribute my success in endurance sports to both improvements in my training and to further improvements in my race nutrition.

About the Book

The sport of triathlon has exploded in recent years. In 2009, more than 1.2 million Americans completed at least one triathlon. Maybe you were one of those 1.2 million, or maybe you are currently training for your very first triathlon. Whatever your experience in the sport of triathlon, or lack thereof, this book will help you improve your everyday nutrition as well as your training and race-related sports nutrition.

It is crucial that every triathlete has a solid knowledge base in nutrition. Now, if you've never paid much attention to nutrition before, you may be less than confident in your abilities to understand how nutrients affect both your health and athletic performance. That is where this book comes in.

There are three different sections in the pages that follow. The first teaches you about nutrition basics, and what nutrients you need to eat on a daily basis in order to ensure a balanced, healthy diet that is specific to triathletes. This nutrient-focused section lays the groundwork for the rest of the book.

Once your everyday dietary needs are taken care of, you can focus on training and race-specific nutrition. The second section of this book addresses exactly that. The sport of triathlon is unique because races vary from relatively short distances to ultra-endurance-race distances. Nutritional needs for each of these races will vary. Therefore, this section includes distance-specific chapters covering the four common distances of triathlon: Sprint, Olympic, half Ironman, and full Ironman.

The final section is much like a troubleshooting guide, addressing questions frequently asked by triathletes—including travel concerns, supplements, weight management, and dealing with injury—some or all of which I'm certain will apply to you, as well. We will sort through these common issues and give you the tools you need to address them, and others.

Once you master these sections, it's time to apply what you have learned. Included (starting on page 162) are sample meal plans and race- and training-specific nutrition plans you can use to get started. Examples of these race and training nutrition plans cover four different race distances:

Sprint, Olympic, half Ironman, and full Ironman. Additionally, the daily meal plans are created for four different-size triathletes, two men and two women. Finally, this section of the book contains common sports nutrition products to help guide you when you are designing your very own nutrition plan. Because there are a number of terms or abbreviations you may not be familiar with, the appendix includes a glossary of terms for things that may not be clearly defined in the book, along with a list of defined abbreviations.

Mastering the Essentials

Before we dive in to part one, there are some basic nutrition concepts I want to introduce you to here. There are six essential nutrients that we will discuss in the following chapters. An essential nutrient is one that your body requires to function properly. These nutrients must come from your diet, since your body does not synthesize these nutrients in sufficient quantities (or, in some cases, doesn't produce them at all). These nutrients include your macronutrients (carbohydrates, fats, and proteins), micronutrients (vitamins and minerals), and water.

It is important to understand that the food you eat contains energy. This energy, which is converted into chemical energy in the body, is described to you in terms of calories. Therefore, the food you eat (which contains calories) is converted into energy in the body. This energy is used to help your body function, and to allow you to be able to perform physical activity or exercise. When this energy is used by the body, we say it is expended energy, and we also measure this in calories. You will see reference to this as we discuss and calculate caloric intake throughout the book.

So, why do you need to know this? Well, the six categories of nutrients are important for a triathlete, and a deficiency in any one of these six nutrients can, and will, hinder performance. While you should be mindful of all of these essential nutrients, for you triathletes, the three most important nutritional considerations are carbohydrates, electrolytes (specifically, sodium), and fluids. The "Big Three," as I call them (carbohydrates, electrolytes, and fluids), are key to a successful training and race-nutrition plan. So,

Make Note: The Big Three (carbohydrates, electrolytes, and fluids) are key to a successful training and race-nutrition plan.

if you need to narrow your focus or simplify your nutrition plan, focus on the Big Three.

I offer recommendations on nutrient intake throughout this book, and you'll note that some sections provide very detailed information, while other sections have more-broad recommendations. But don't you worry—I'll walk you through all of this. Start with the general recommendations, and after you feel like you have a good understanding of those, then focus on the more-detailed aspects of your sports-nutrition diet.

> **Make Note:** Working out your nutrition also means occasionally working with some numbers and percentages. To make things easier for the math-challenged, I include several resources throughout this book to help you with your nutrition plan for everyday living, training, and racing.

Most nutrient-intake recommendations that are based on body weight use kilograms instead of pounds. This is because the scientific community (where the research is done to determine these recommendations) uses kilograms rather than pounds. Therefore, you first need to be able to convert your body weight from pounds to kilograms. There are 2.2 pounds for every kilogram. So, to figure out your kilogram weight, here's the formula you use:

Your body weight (in pounds) _____
divided by 2.2 = _____ kg

If your new body weight in kilograms isn't slightly less than half of your body weight in pounds, then you did something wrong. For example, if you weigh 130 pounds, your body weight in kilograms is 59. (Doesn't that sound better, anyway?)

Additionally, nutritionists regularly use a lot of different abbreviations. Since you will come across some of them in this book, I have included a list of common abbreviations in the appendix (see page 159).

Monitoring and Maintaining a Healthy Diet

While most of this book focuses on specific nutrition recommendations for triathletes, I also touch upon maintaining a healthy diet (and, truthfully, the everyday diet for a triathlete is not that different from a healthy diet for the general public). If you follow the recommendations suggested in this book, you will be consuming a well-balanced diet that should improve your overall health and well-being. Nearly every chapter in this book has nutrient recommendations in it that will hopefully inspire you to make some changes in your diet.

Before you can change your diet, you need to know what you currently eat. Closer scrutiny can show that what is sometimes thought of as a poor diet may actually be surprisingly healthy, while conversely, a diet that is perceived as healthy isn't quite as healthy as you may think. In either case, there may be room for improvement.

I highly recommend that you record your food and fluid intake for several days before trying to change your diet. This means paying close attention to the nutrients and calories you put into your body. You can figure out the amount of carbohydrates, protein, and fat—as well as how many total calories—are in your diet based on food labels, or by researching specific product nutritional information, or you can use a program that will analyze all of your food for you.

One recommended program is MyPlate (choosemyplate.gov), which is free and fairly user-friendly. You can use the SuperTracker function on this website to input your food and fluid intake each day. This can be a little time-consuming at first, but if you are like most people, some of the foods you eat one day will be repeated at different times during the week.

For example, maybe you eat a bowl of oatmeal for breakfast each day. Well, once you put in the information for that oatmeal one time, it will be there with one click of the button for subsequent days. The benefits of using a program such as MyPlate is that it tells you your nutrient totals (which are not always easy to calculate from food labels, especially your micronutrients) at the end of the day, and whether or not you met your nutrient needs (such as total calories; carbohydrate, fat, and protein intake; micronutrient intake; and fluid intake). Once you know what you currently consume, the recommendations in this book will be easier to follow and will set you up for success.

If I had read a book like this one before my first marathon at age eighteen, I think I would have prepared myself for a much faster (and less painful) race. I don't know what the outcome might have been with proper nutrition, but I did learn that I never wanted to look back at a race again with regrets about any of the nutrition decisions I had made. I now know what I need to be doing so I can practice optimal nutrition every time I leave my house for a training session. My goal is that at the end of every race, I can confidently say that I had great race nutrition, and that it helped me to finish strong.

By the end of this book, I hope you'll be able to say the same thing!

Part One:
The Triathlete's Diet—
The Essential Nutrients

Before you can create and tailor a specific diet for your racing and training needs, you first need to have a solid nutrition knowledge base and a healthy day-to-day diet. In this section we'll cover the basics and the essential facts you need to know about nutrition. Consider this the groundwork for the rest of the book. Here we'll discuss your necessary macronutrients (carbohydrates, proteins, and fats), as well as the vitamins, minerals, and fluids necessary to maintain a healthy diet.

It can actually be more challenging to master your everyday nutrition than it can be to master your race and training nutrition. However, your training and race-day nutrition will only work if you eat a healthy diet on a daily basis. Consider your everyday nutrition the foundation or base of a pyramid. You have to have a strong foundation before you can add more layers to the pyramid. A weak foundation affects everything else. Once you have the basics mastered, then you can start thinking about nutrition for training and racing.

CHAPTER 1

Carbohydrates

I used to coach a triathlete (we'll call him Bob) who wanted to lose weight. He decided to go on the low-carbohydrate Atkins Diet because he had not been successful in his previous attempts to lose weight. Despite my objections to this diet for an endurance athlete, Bob pursued this plan. Within a week, he was experiencing headaches and feeling tired, lethargic, and irritable. He hadn't had a good training session since he'd started the low-carb diet. For any endurance athlete (and that includes all distances of triathlons), remember this: Carbohydrates are your friend, not your enemy.

Let me start by saying this: "Low-carb diet" and "triathlete" should never exist in the same sentence. I don't care what your friends have told you about how much weight they lost or how they have adjusted to a low-carbohydrate intake. As a triathlete, carbohydrates are your best friend. They are the most important source of energy, and you will not train or perform at your highest level without adequate carbohydrates in the diet.

When you think of carbohydrates, you should think of fuel for your body. Carbohydrates are macronutrients, which means they provide a lot of energy, and your body needs them in large quantities in order to function properly. Carbohydrates are made up of carbon, hydrogen, and oxygen molecules, and are the primary source of fuel or energy (calories) for your body. Having adequate carbohydrates—and the right kind—in your diet are important for optimal health and athletic performance. Each gram of carbohydrates provides 4 calories of energy.

Types of Carbohydrates

There are two types of carbohydrates: simple and complex. Simple carbohydrates include your simple sugars (also known as monosaccharides and disaccharides). The three most common monosaccharides in our diet are:

1. Glucose

2. Fructose

3. Galactose

Glucose is the most prevalent of these simple sugars and is found in nearly any product that contains simple sugars. This is because glucose is part of sucrose (which is table sugar, covered in more detail below). Therefore, all sports-nutrition products, sports drinks, sodas, and candy contain glucose. Fructose, as the name implies, is found primarily in fruit and is known as fruit sugar. It is also the sweetest of the three monosaccharides. Galactose is not very prevalent in the average diet and usually only exists as part of lactose (see below), which is a milk sugar found in all dairy products.

This brings us to your other simple carbohydrates, the disaccharides. Disaccharides are two simple sugars combined together. The most prevalent in our diet are:

1. Sucrose = Glucose + Fructose

2. Lactose = Glucose + Galactose

3. Maltose = Glucose + Glucose

Sucrose is simply table sugar, and it is so sweet because of the combination of glucose and fructose. Lactose is milk sugar and is found in all dairy products. Some athletes are lactose-intolerant, a term that is often misconstrued. (Note that this is not an allergy to lactose; rather, it is the inability of the body to digest lactose properly.) People who consume dairy products and are lactose-intolerant will usually end up getting mild to severe gastrointestinal (GI) distress. Therefore, athletes who are even slightly lactose-intolerant should avoid dairy products in the hours leading up to a race, and they also need to be careful of dairy intake on a daily basis. Maltose, which is simply two glucose molecules combined together, is quite rare in our diets; in fact, we don't really eat foods with maltose in them. When we eat foods that contain starch, it is eventually broken down into maltose in our bodies.

As far as athletes are concerned, glucose will be the primary source of sugar in their diet, along with some fructose.

Your complex carbohydrates contain three or more sugar molecules linked together and are mainly in the form of starches or fiber. When you eat starches, they are broken down into simple sugars (most of which will be glucose) by your digestive system and are then absorbed into the body as simple sugars. Complex carbohydrates (starches, fiber) should make up the majority of your carbohydrate sources, and simple carbohydrates (simple sugars) should be a much smaller percentage of your total carbohydrate intake.

Importance of Fiber

Fiber is an important component of a healthy diet. There are two types of fiber that you can obtain from your diet: soluble and insoluble fibers. Your soluble fibers are found primarily in oats, barley, legumes (dried beans, peas, lentils), and some fruits and vegetables. Insoluble fiber sources include whole-grain products, nuts, seeds, and some vegetables. While each type of fiber provides different health benefits for the body, in general, fiber increases satiety (feelings of fullness), decreases cholesterol levels, helps regulate blood glucose levels, prevents and treats constipation, and may decrease your risk of developing colon cancer. The recommendations for daily fiber intake are 30 to 38 grams per day for men and 21 to 25 grams per day for women. Unfortunately, average US intake is about 10 to 20 grams per day—in some cases, less than half the recommended amount.

Triathletes should try to meet the recommended daily intakes for fiber, but I do want to point out one thing: Much of the fiber you consume in your diet is non-digestible, which means that your body cannot break it down into simple sugars for absorption. As a result, it can cause some GI disturbances. Therefore, if you have a low fiber intake right now, you should gradually increase the amount of fiber in your diet rather than making drastic increases, in order to ease your body into it. I recommend that you shy away from a high-fiber diet in the twenty-four hours leading up to a race to prevent possible GI problems during the race. We will discuss specific dietary needs further in part two (see page 55) as part of the pre-race nutrition information.

Functions of Carbohydrates in the Body

When the carbohydrates you eat are digested (aka, broken down into simple sugars), they are absorbed from the GI tract into the bloodstream (mainly as glucose). Your body maintains a fairly constant, yet small, amount of glucose in the blood. The remaining glucose is either metabolized or stored. If it is metabolized (meaning, used up by the body) right away, it immediately provides energy for the body. If it is stored, it's important to remember that there is a limit on the storage capacity in your body; once that storage capacity has reached its maximum level, "overflow" glucose is converted into fatty acids and stored in fat tissue. The storage form of glucose is called glycogen, which is stored only in liver and muscle cells.

As I mentioned above, carbohydrates are the primary energy source for the body. Virtually all cells in the body use carbohydrates for energy, and some tissues (such as the brain and central nervous system) rely on carbohydrates almost solely for energy. During exercise, you use mostly carbohydrates and fat for energy (only small amounts of protein are used). The higher the intensity of exercise, the greater the reliance on carbohydrates to fuel that exercise. For triathletes, who expend a large amount of energy, this means that the carbohydrates are an important nutrient.

Common Food Sources

It is pretty easy to get enough carbohydrates in your diet. Just about everywhere you turn, you will find carbohydrates. So many foods in our diets contain carbohydrates: grains, breads, cereals, fruits, vegetables, desserts, candy, beverages, etc. (The list goes on and on.) In fact, it is much harder to go on a low-carb diet than it is to increase the amount of carbohydrates you eat on a daily basis, because food items become so restricted. People who go on low-carb diets usually end up losing weight, but it's not because of eating less carbohydrates; it's simply due to the fact that so many foods are restricted from their diet that they eat fewer calories each day.

A lot of today's diet recommendations make sugar out to be the bad guy, something to avoid at all costs. While it's true that high sugar consumption does tend to lead to weight gain and health problems—if the high consumption occurs for long periods of time, in conjunction with sedentary lifestyles—it's also true that as a triathlete, sugar is sometimes your best friend. (We will discuss this in detail in part two of this book.) Rather than cutting out certain nutrients or sugars entirely, the goal is to eat healthier, complex carbohydrates for the majority of your day, and then focus on those simple sugars during and immediately after exercise (more to come on this in part two, page 55).

Common food sources for complex carbohydrates (starches and fibers) include anything with grains (such as cereals, oatmeal, bread, tortillas, and rice), pastas, legumes (beans), fruits, and vegetables. Some common food sources for simple sugars include desserts, candy, sweetened beverages (soda, Gatorade, lemonade), and just about anything else you can think of that is sweet and does not contain artificial sweeteners. For triathletes, you will also find simple sugars in gels, bars, Jelly Belly Sport Beans, Clif Shot Bloks (just a few of the many sports nutrition products commonly used by endurance athletes), and most other products that are marketed for consumption during exercise.

What Is the Glycemic Index?

The glycemic index was developed to determine how different carbohydrates affect blood sugar (glucose) levels. Knowing the glycemic index of certain foods and understanding what the glycemic index is will help you as you choose foods for a healthy everyday diet. It will also help you when you are choosing foods for pre- and post-training (you will find recommendations for either low- or high-glycemic-index foods in part two of this book). The glycemic index assigns a number to each food based on how quickly it leads to increases in blood glucose levels, with a value of 100 being the highest (pure glucose). Carbohydrates that are digested and absorbed more quickly (such as simple sugars) have a higher glycemic index than those carbohydrates that are more slowly digested and absorbed (such as complex carbohydrates). Carbohydrates with a high glycemic index will most rapidly increase blood glucose levels.

So how do the glycemic index values translate? A food that has a high glycemic index will have a value of 70 or greater, while a moderate-glycemic-index food will have values between 56 and 69, and low-glycemic-index foods will have values of 55 or less. Typically, foods with a large amount of simple sugars have high glycemic indexes. However, the amount of fat and protein also affects the glycemic index of foods. Foods with more fat and/or protein slow down the digestion and absorption of nutrients, so even high-sugar foods (such as a Snickers bar) can have a low glycemic index because of the amount of fat and protein in the product. Below is a chart listing the glycemic index of some common foods.

GLYCEMIC INDEX OF SOME COMMON FOODS

LOW GLYCEMIC INDEX (≤55)	MODERATE GLYCEMIC INDEX (56–69)	HIGH GLYCEMIC INDEX (≥70)
Orange juice–52	Rye bread–64	Waffles–76
Whole-grain bread–50	Pineapple–66	Baguette–95
Brown rice–55	Mangos–56	White bread–71
Low-fat yogurt–33	Raisins–64	Bagels–72
Banana–54	Sweet corn–56	Pretzels–81
Orange–44	Pita bread–57	Corn chips–74
Apple–38	Taco shells–68	Watermelon–72
Sweet potato–54	Couscous–61	Cheerios–74
Most vegetables–15 to 50	Cornmeal–68	French fries–75
Whole-grain pasta–45	Ice cream (full-fat)–61	Graham crackers–74
Black beans (boiled)–30	Mac and cheese–64	Dried dates–70
Spaghetti (white, cooked)–38	Muffins–65	Raisin Bran–73
Milk (skim)–32	Wheat Thins crackers–67	Baked potato–85
Snickers bar–41	White rice–64	Vanilla wafers–77
All-Bran–51	Power bars–58	Gatorade–78

Source: Information for this table obtained from DRI reports (nap.edu), Institute of Medicine of the National Academies.

So here's why all of this glycemic-index talk is important for you: For general health (and especially for people with type 2 diabetes), I recommend you eat foods with low to moderate glycemic indexes and minimize the amount of high-glycemic-index foods eaten. As a triathlete, while you should eat low- to moderate-glycemic-index foods as part of your everyday diet, this will change during training sessions or races.

During exercise, you want to supply your body with carbohydrates as quickly as possible so they can immediately supply the body with energy. Therefore, I recommend the intake of high-glycemic-index foods during exercise. Similarly, it is important to replenish carbohydrate stores (glycogen) as quickly as possible after exercise. Therefore, I also recommend high-glycemic-index foods right after exercise. These are probably the only two instances where an athlete should try to eat high-glycemic-index foods. Before exercise, and throughout the rest of the day, low- to moderate-glycemic-index foods are best. I will refer to the glycemic index quite frequently in part two as we delve more deeply into specific triathlete races (see page 72).

Carbohydrate Recommendations

General Population Recommendations: There are various recommendations designed to help all of us eat a healthy, balanced diet and to provide our bodies with everything they need. One of these recommendations is called the acceptable macronutrient distribution range (AMDR), which is basically the "acceptable" amount or range of a nutrient that we should try to get in our diets. The AMDR for carbohydrates is 45 to 65 percent of your daily caloric intake. The amount of carbohydrates needed to supply the brain with glucose is 130 grams per day. That is the amount needed just to supply the brain—that is to say, just to keep you thinking straight. Therefore, your actual intake should be higher than that to provide adequate amounts in order for the entire body to function properly.

Of those total calories coming from carbohydrates (45 to 65 percent), half that amount should come from complex carbohydrates, such as those found in grains (cereals, oatmeal, bread, tortillas, and rice), pastas, legumes (beans), fruits, and vegetables. Added sugar to foods should also be limited. To follow a healthy diet, you should eat plenty of vegetables, fruits, and whole grains while consuming sugar only in moderation.

Triathlete Recommendations: As a triathlete, you're expending lots of energy swimming, biking, and running regularly. As a result, you may need more carbohydrates in your diet than the average person. This is especially true if you put in a lot of training hours or do a great deal of endurance training (two-plus hours per day of training). If you fall into this category, I recommend you get 5 to 10 grams of carbohydrates per kilogram of body weight. The more endurance training you do, the higher you will be on that range. As a general rule, if you are training for a half or full Ironman, then you should intake 8 to 10 grams per kilogram of body weight. If you are training for a sprint or Olympic distance race, then you can intake around 6 to 8 grams per kilogram of body weight. Again, we'll dive into this more specifically in part two (see page 56).

Make Note: The recommended intake for triathletes is 5 to 10 grams of carbohydrate per kilogram of body weight. Those triathletes training for Sprint and Olympic distance races should be at around 6 to 8 grams per kilogram of body weight, while triathletes training for a half or full Ironman should be at the upper end of that range (8 to 10 grams per kilogram of body weight).

The above range of recommendations usually corresponds to about 50 to 65 percent of total calories coming from carbohydrates (not unlike the recommendations for the general public). However, for those of you training for a half or full Ironman who are eating 8 to 10 grams per kilogram of body weight, you may be as high as 75 percent of total calories from carbohydrates. This is okay, but don't go any higher than this percentage. Anything above 75 percent of calories from carbohydrates, and you will not get enough fat and/or protein in your diet. It's important to maintain balance in your diet, so follow those percentages.

Calculating Carbohydrate Intake

Let me guess—you just saw the word calculate, and some of you are now freaking out. I know it can be intimidating to read through these number and percentage recommendations, but never fear, I'll walk you through it. Even those of us who are math-challenged can do this! In the sidebar on page 11 is an example of how to calculate the total grams (and calories) of carbohydrates needed on a daily basis, based on these recommendations. Before you look at that sidebar, here is a description of the steps involved in this calculation:

1. You will first need to calculate your weight in kilograms, so see page 12 for a refresher on that equation.

2. Identify the range of grams of carbohydrates per kilogram of body weight based off of the race you're running (see page 9 for a refresher).

3. Multiply your kilogram weight by the recommended grams of carbohydrates. (Note: If the recommended amount is a range, choose from within that range.)

4. Since there are 4 calories for each gram of carbohydrate, multiply the number you got in step three by 4 to get your total calories of carbohydrates daily.

5. Take your answer from step four and divide it by the total number of daily calories you are consuming to give you the percentage of calories that are coming from carbohydrates. This step is done to make sure the gram amount you choose still fits within the recommended percentages.

Once you figure out the amount of carbohydrates you need, check to see if it falls within the 50 to 75 percent range of carbohydrates for the diet. For example, if you chose 10 grams of carbohydrates per kilogram of body weight and it ends up being 80 percent of your total daily calories, then you should adjust to 8 or 9 grams of carbohydrates per kilogram of body weight. Conversely, if you choose 7 grams of carbohydrates per kilogram of body weight and it ends up being 40 percent of your total daily calories, then you need to raise the carbohydrate intake. In some cases, when total caloric intake is quite high, 10 grams of carbohydrates per kilogram of body weight will not be enough to fall within the 50 to 75 percent recommended range. In those

CALCULATING RECOMMENDED DAILY CARBOHYDRATE NEEDS: An Example

A person (125.4 pounds) who is training for a half Ironman needs 8 to 10 grams of carbohydrates per kilogram of body weight.

1. Body weight: 125.4 divided by 2.2 = 57 kilograms.
2. We will use 8 grams of carbohydrates per kilogram of body weight for this triathlete.
3. 57 kilograms x 8 grams = 456 grams of carbohydrate daily.
4. This equates to 1,824 calories of carbohydrates daily (456 grams x 4 calories per gram for carbohydrates = 1,824 calories).
5. If this person eats 2,700 calories per day, this equates to 68 percent of calories coming from carbohydrates (1,824 divided by 2,700 = 0.68, or 68 percent).

The recommended intake is to get somewhere between 50 to 75 percent of total calories coming from carbohydrates. The calculation in our example has 68 percent of calories coming from carbohydrates, which means it falls within the recommended range. Therefore, 8 grams of carbohydrates per kilogram of body weight on a daily basis is an appropriate recommendation for this athlete.

extreme cases, you may have to go as high as 12 grams of carbohydrates per kilogram of body weight. However, this usually occurs only with very high volumes of training (such as five to seven hours per day of exercise).

Now you can calculate your own intake. Remember that there are 2.2 pounds per kilogram, so take your weight in pounds and divide it by 2.2 to get your weight in kilograms.

Here's how to do your own calculation:

1. Your weight in pounds divided by 2.2 to get weight in kilograms = _____ .

2. Choose the gram amount of carbohydrates from the recommendations: _____ .

3. Your weight (in kilograms): _____ x 8 grams[1]
   = _____ grams of carbohydrate daily.

4. Equates to _____ calories of carbohydrate daily
   (_____ grams x 4 calories per gram for carbohydrate).

5. If you eat _____ calories per day, this equates to _____ percent of calories coming from carbohydrates (total calories of carbohydrate daily divided by total daily calories = _____ percent).

Congratulations—you've survived the math! Phew! Now you know how much carbohydrates you should consume each day. It may seem cumbersome to add up the grams of carbohydrates that you consume each day, but if you do this for one week, you will have a very good idea of the amount of carbohydrates you eat on a daily basis, and which foods (and amounts of those foods) will get you to the appropriate levels.

Carbohydrate Loading

Carbohydrate loading, which is the process of storing extra amounts of carbohydrates in the body, tends to be more popular among marathoners than triathletes, but the benefits can apply to any athlete who exercises for more than two hours. Note that some people call this glycogen loading instead of carbohydrate loading. Glycogen is simply the name of the storage form of carbohydrate in the body. Both terms mean exactly the same thing.

Here's the science behind carbohydrate loading: Your muscles have a limited amount of glycogen (storage form of carbohydrate) that they can keep or store. Once your glycogen stores are depleted, your performance will suffer. The more glycogen you can store prior to an event, the more fuel you will be able to utilize during your race. If you race for two hours or less,

---

1 Note: You can replace the 8 grams in your own calculation with a different number based on the race you are training for.

you won't deplete your glycogen stores, so carbohydrate loading is unnecessary. However, for longer races, if you can trick your body into storing more glycogen than usual, you may be able to perform better. Thus, for triathletes, carbohydrate loading is most beneficial for the half Ironman and Ironman distances, and possibly even for Olympic distance races.

Here are the steps to carbohydrate loading:

1. Seven days prior to the event, you should perform a long, strenuous workout in order to deplete muscle glycogen stores. This workout needs to be of moderate intensity for two-plus hours, or high intensity for at least ninety minutes.

2. This is followed by three days of a low- to moderate-carbohydrate diet, where approximately 35 to 50 percent of total calories should come from carbohydrates. During this time, you should decrease the amount of exercise you do.

3. For the next three days you need to consume a high-carbohydrate diet, where up to 75 percent of your total calories should come from carbohydrates, and further decrease the amount of exercise you do.

4. The seventh and final day of carbohydrate loading is your competition day. On this day, you should follow the recommendations for the twenty-four hours leading up to your specific event, which will be outlined later in this book (see part two, starting on page 55).

So why follow these specific steps? Step one is necessary in order to deplete glycogen stores in the muscle. Your body then responds by trying to replenish those stores as quickly as possible. This is where step two comes in. By depriving your body of adequate carbohydrates, it cannot replenish glycogen stores. This causes an adaptation in the body. Your body is very smart, and to compensate it will increase the enzyme (which is protein that helps reactions occur) activity that makes and stores glycogen in muscles. By the time your body has increased those enzymes—it typically takes up to three days to maximize enzyme activity—you reach step three. During this step, the high-carb diet provides all the glycogen necessary to store even more carbohydrates in the muscle than if you had never deprived it of carbo-hydrates in the first place.

The end result? After this seven-day carbohydrate-loading regime, you will have more glycogen stored in muscle than if you had just been following your regular diet for that week leading up to your race. One caveat: It is really important to remember that you have to decrease your exercise volume (both in intensity and in duration) throughout that seven-day regimen. If you don't, you will use up that glycogen during each workout, particularly in step three, and thus won't be able to super-load the muscles with glycogen.

At this point you may be wondering, "Why wouldn't every athlete carbohydrate-load before their Olympic distance or half Ironman races?" The answer is that there are some drawbacks to carbohydrate loading. First of all, it doesn't work for everyone. You can try it once and if it doesn't seem to work for you, or if you don't like the other side effects, then it's probably not something you want to repeat for your next race. Second, when you store glycogen, you store water along with it. In fact, you store 3 grams of water for every 1 gram of carbohydrate you store. This means that water weight gain can occur in the days leading up to a race, which some athletes don't like because they think the extra water weight actually slows them down. Third, if you are used to a fairly high-carbohydrate diet (which you should be as a triathlete), then lowering your carbohydrate intake for three days dur-ing step two can sometimes cause fatigue, headaches, and irritability. This may not be exactly how you want to feel in the days leading up to your race. Finally, some people don't like decreasing their exercise volume to the extent necessary in order to store extra glycogen.

There are two sides to every argument, and you have to experiment a little to see what works best for you. I personally like to glycogen-load before marathons and half Ironman races (and my best times seem to coincide with the races that I chose to carbohydrate-load), although I have not tried it before a full Ironman race. It seems that with races of such long distances, the carbohydrates you take in during the race are more important than stor-ing some extra glycogen beforehand. Even if you carbohydrate-load before an Ironman race, you will be glycogen-depleted before you finish the race.

There are a few different methods of carbohydrate loading, but research shows that they all produce similar results. The main difference between the methods comes during step two, the depletion phase. Some older methods recommend a low-carbohydrate diet (10 to 35 percent of total calories), while some newer methods recommend a moderate amount of carbohydrates during step two (35 to 50 percent of total calories). Most methods seem to yield similar results, so if you don't want to drastically cut your carbohydrate intake during step two, you can achieve the same results with modest decreases in the carbohydrate content of your diet.

I have used a couple of different methods of carbohydrate loading, and I can personally attest to how difficult it is to drastically change my carbohydrate intake (from 70 down to 20 percent). Consider your family and friends when choosing your method; my husband and coworkers would most certainly vote for me to follow a more-moderate cut in carbohydrates to reduce irritability and crabbiness!

If carbohydrate loading seems like too much of a burden, or if it seems like it would be too difficult to count up your carbs for the week before a race, you can instead try to eat a low-carb diet during step two and a high-carb diet during step three. The percentages of calories coming from carbohydrates may not be exactly right, but you will likely get the benefits of storing extra glycogen in your muscles.

CHAPTER 2

Protein

Like dietary carbohydrates, protein is also an essential macronutrient. This means your body must have it to function properly, and it provides energy (calories). In fact, you get the same number of calories from each gram of protein that you do from carbohydrates (4 calories per gram). However, the functions of protein are quite different from carbohydrates. Whereas carbs are your body's primary energy source, protein contributes very little to energy production. Only about 5 to 10 percent (and sometimes as high as 15 percent during ultra-endurance events) of all the calories you burn each day come from protein.

Rather than being used to produce energy, protein is instead reserved for other important functions that no other nutrient can do. This includes the building and repairing of tissues (skeletal muscle, bones, ligaments, tendons, organs, etc). Protein is also used to make many hormones in your body, such as insulin, and it makes antibodies that destroy bacteria and viruses. Additionally, protein is used to make enzymes; it acts as a transporter in the blood and tissues; and it helps with fluid balance. In short, protein is necessary in order for nearly every system in the body to function properly.

Protein is particularly critical for you, the triathlete, because you constantly do damage to your body's tissues, which then need to be repaired, or sometimes built anew.

Types of Protein

The protein in your food is made up of amino acids (AAs) that are linked together. In fact, each protein that you eat usually contains several hundred AAs. As you eat those proteins, digestive enzymes break them down into individual AAs, which are then absorbed into the bloodstream. Once in your bloodstream, AAs are synthesized (or manufactured) into different proteins, depending on what your body needs. For example, some of those AAs may be used to repair damaged skeletal muscle, while others may be used to make antibodies or hormones, and still others may be used for energy.

Unlike carbohydrates and fats, you cannot store excess protein in the body. While you do have an AA "pool"—which is basically a certain number of AAs that circulate in your bloodstream and are available for whatever protein your body needs—you do not store excess AAs as protein. Instead, any excess protein that you eat gets converted into fat and stored in the body. Yup, that's right. Your body is very efficient at storing fat. Any excess carbohydrates, proteins, or fats all end up getting stored as fat. If you continually eat too much carbohydrate, fat, or protein, you will gain weight from the extra fat you store. Also, since you cannot store excess protein in the body, it is important to get the recommended amount in your diet on a daily basis.

I mentioned that AAs are combined to make proteins. While there are tons of different kinds of proteins, there are only twenty AAs that exist in our food supply; nine of those AAs are essential, and eleven are nonessential. This means that your body can make eleven of those AAs, but the other nine must come from your diet. Now, you may wonder why this is important for you. Well, to recover properly after training or racing, you need to make sure you get all nine of your essential AAs so that repair and synthesis of tissues can take place.

The table below shows you which AAs are essential and which are nonessential. Now, before you start worrying that you need to learn and remember all of these AAs, let me reassure you: You basically need to know which types of foods contain all of your essential AAs, and then you'll know that your bases are covered. A complete protein is one that contains all nine of your essential AAs. Any animal protein (meat, eggs, and dairy) is a complete protein. Incomplete proteins are missing at least one essential AA. All plant proteins, with the exception of soy, are incomplete proteins. That's not to say that plant proteins are bad; you just need to make sure you get the correct combination of plant proteins in order to get all nine of your essential AAs.

> **Make Note:** There are both essential and nonessential amino acids. A complete protein contains all nine essential amino acids. All animal proteins and soy are complete proteins. All other plant proteins are incomplete proteins (missing at least one essential amino acid).

In other words, you want your incomplete proteins to complement one another. For example, grains are often missing lysine (an AA), so they match up well with legumes, which have a lot of lysine. In general, grains match up well with legumes, and legumes match up well with nuts and seeds. Remember that soy is the only plant protein that does contain all nine essential AAs.

ESSENTIAL AMINO ACIDS (EAAs)	NONESSENTIAL AMINO ACIDS (NEAAs)
Phenylalanine	Alanine
Valine	Aspartic Acid
Tryptophan	Asparagine
Threonine	Glutamic Acid
Isoleucine	Glutamine
Methionine	Glycine
Histidine	Serine
Leucine	Arginine
Lysine	Proline
	Cysteine
	Tyrosine

Food Sources of Protein

There are two main sources of protein in your diet—animal and plant. Animal sources and soy are complete proteins, whereas all other plant sources are incomplete proteins. For animal sources, foods rich in protein include meats (chicken, turkey, fish, beef, pork, lamb, etc.), dairy products, and eggs. The richest sources of plant protein tend to be legumes (beans), nuts and seeds, and tofu. The table below lists food sources that are protein-rich. You'll notice plant proteins on this chart; simply because they are missing at least one essential AA does not disqualify them from serving as good, healthy options. Don't be fooled into thinking that animal proteins are better for you because they are complete. Animal proteins are often high in fat (especially saturated fats, which are not heart-healthy) and cholesterol. Therefore, plant proteins are often a healthier choice to add to your diet. When laying out your meal plans, try to get a mixture of plant proteins and lean animal proteins in your diet.

PRODUCT	GRAMS	PRODUCT	GRAMS
Meat, Fish, and Soy		**Beans and Seeds**	
Chicken breast (4 oz)	35g	Black beans (1 cup)	15g
Cod fillet (4 oz.)	20g	Black-eyed peas (1 cup)	11g
Ham deli meat (4 oz.)	19g	Chickpeas (garbanzo beans) (1 cup)	12g
Hamburger patty (4 oz.)	28g	Soybeans, cooked (1 cup)	29g
Lamb chop (4 oz.)	20g	Kidney beans (1 cup)	13g
Pork chop (4 oz.)	77g	Lentils (1 cup)	18g
Salmon fillet (4 oz.)	22g	Lima beans (1 cup)	10g
Tofu (4 oz.)	8g	Peas (1 cup)	9g
Turkey breast (4 oz.)	20g	Pinto beans (1 cup)	14g
Turkey deli meat (4 oz.)	22g	Pumpkin seeds (½ cup)	6g
Dairy		**Nuts and Protein Powders**	
Cheese (1 slice)	6g	Almonds, whole (1 cup)	30g
Cottage Cheese (1 cup)	28g	Walnut halves, shelled (1 cup)	15g
Eggs (1 large egg)	6g	Peanut butter (2 tbsp)	8g
Milk (1 cup)	8g	Peanuts (1 cup)	37g
Yogurt (1 cup)	12g	Soy or whey protein (1 scoop)	23g

Protein Powders

There is a huge market for protein powders, protein shakes/drinks, and protein bars. These are usually more popular among strength athletes, but triathletes often supplement their diet with some of these products, as well. Whether or not you use them is really personal preference. Some people do not have the time or desire to prepare food to be eaten before and after their workouts, so they like the convenience that these products offer, not to mention the fact that many are chock-full of an array of micronutrients (vitamins and minerals). On the other hand, these products are usually more expensive than food you could prepare yourself, and often contain protein in much higher quantities than is actually necessary.

The most commonly used proteins in these store-bought products are whey, soy, and casein. Egg protein can also be used, but it's not as popular as the other three. Whey protein is derived from milk protein. It is the most popular source of protein in supplements and is digested and absorbed faster than other proteins. Casein protein is also derived from milk protein but is slower-acting; it tends to stimulate protein synthesis to a lesser extent than whey protein, but unlike whey, casein also appears to decrease protein breakdown. Soy protein is derived from soybeans and contains strong antioxidants. Although more research is needed in this area, scientists believe soy protein may actually decrease the risk of developing cardiovascular disease and cancer. Whey, soy, and casein are complete (meaning, they contain all nine EAAs). Some people prefer to buy products that use a combination of these proteins rather than just one type of protein. If you decide to use some of these products, the type you choose is really up to you.

General Protein Recommendations for Adults and for Triathletes

I usually get asked two questions regarding protein intake for athletes. The first question is, "How much protein should I eat?" The second question is, "Should I eat protein before or after I work out?" In answering these questions, I will assume you are a well-rounded triathlete and that you do some weight or resistance training. I assume that your weight training is not designed to help you bulk up (put on huge amounts of muscle mass); rather, I'm guessing you are trying to maintain muscle mass, prevent muscle imbalances and injuries, and improve efficiency and economy of movement. I assume all of this because the protein recommendations that I give here are geared toward endurance athletes, not strength athletes.

There is a lot of contradictory information about how much protein a triathlete actually needs. One of the reasons for all the confusion is that protein recommendations are provided in two different formats. The first is given as a percentage of total calories from protein, and the second is given as recommended grams of protein per kilogram of body weight. We will cover both formats here so that there is no confusion. For protein there is an acceptable macronutrient distribution range (AMDR) of 10 to 35 percent of total calories from protein, with 35 percent being a little on the high side. Sedentary individuals actually need about 12 to 15 percent of calories from protein, whereas endurance athletes (that's you!) need about 15 to 20 percent of total calories from protein. And, yes, despite the training you do, the percentage is not much higher for endurance athletes than it is for sedentary individuals. Keep in mind, though, that as a triathlete you should consume more total calories than a sedentary person, so your absolute amount of protein (total grams) will be higher. This is where the second format of protein recommendations comes into play.

The average sedentary individual needs about 0.8 grams of protein per kilogram of body weight. An endurance athlete needs anywhere from 1.2 grams to 2.0 grams of protein per kilogram of body weight. As you can see, the endurance athlete recommendations can be more than twice as high as a sedentary individual when you calculate it as grams per kilogram of body weight.

Make Note: An endurance athlete needs anywhere from 1.2 grams to 2.0 grams of protein per kilogram of body weight. This should equate to about 15 to 20 percent of total calories from protein.

You should calculate your protein needs in grams per kilogram of body weight and then make sure it falls within about 15 to 20 percent of total calories. You may notice that 1.2 to 2.0 grams of protein per kilogram of body weight is quite a wide range. This is because the amount of protein you need depends on a number of different factors. When choosing a gram amount for yourself, keep the following factors in mind:

1. If you do a high volume of training (such as half or full Ironman training), then you will need to be at the higher end of that protein recommendation.

2. If you try to lose weight, you will need to be at the higher end of the recommendation. This may seem counterintuitive, but if you are cutting total calories (which means you are probably cutting some carbohydrates), you will need enough protein for all of the normal functions that protein takes care of, as well as some extra protein that can be converted into carbohydrates (described in more detail later in this chapter on pages 23–24).

3. If you ramp up your training, you will need to be at the higher end of the protein recommendation, because you are likely to do more protein synthesis (tissue repair and building).

4. If you are injured or sick (which is pretty common at some point in time during triathlon training), you will need to be at the higher end of the protein recommendation.

Now, if you do moderate amounts of training (such as for a Sprint or Olympic distance triathlon), you don't suffer from injury, and you aren't changing your body weight, then you can probably be at the low to middle end of that protein-recommendation range.

You should never go above 2 grams of protein per kilogram of body weight. Going higher than that puts additional stress on your body (especially on your kidneys), and usually ends up getting stored as fat. (Remember: You cannot store excess protein.)

Here's how to calculate your daily protein needs:

1. Your body weight (in kilograms) x _____ grams per kilogram = _____ grams of protein daily

2. _____ grams of protein daily x 4 calories per gram = _____ total calories from protein

CALCULATING RECOMMENDED DAILY PROTEIN NEEDS:
An Example

A triathlete weighs 70 kilograms (154 pounds) and is doing Ironman training, while also trying to drop some weight. The lower end of the recommended range (based on his/her circumstances) is:

1. 70 kilograms x 1.7 grams of protein = 119 grams of protein daily.
2. 119 grams of protein x 4 calories per gram = 476 total calories from protein.

The upper end of the recommended range (based on his/her circumstances) is:

1. 70 kilograms x 2.0 grams of protein = 140 grams of protein daily.
2. 140 grams of protein x 4 calories per gram = 560 total calories from protein.

If this athlete consumes 2,800 calories per day, this equates to 17 to 20 percent of total calories coming from protein each day, which fits nicely into the recommended percentages (476 calories divided by 2,800 calories = 0.17, or 17 percent; 560 calories divided by 2,800 calories = 0.2, or 20 percent).

Using Protein to Make Carbohydrates

One unique function of protein is the ability to convert AAs into glucose. This process is called gluconeogenesis, or, the creation of new glucose. (I know—these terms just keep getting crazier and crazier. If you want to sound really smart at your next office party, start throwing around words like glu-coneogenesis; people will either think you're really smart—or really dorky.)

In general, your body does not do a lot of gluconeogenesis. However, when carbohydrates are not readily available (such as during long training sessions or long triathlons without proper nutrition, or when you're on a low-calorie or low-carb diet), you will increase gluconeogenesis. This can be both good and bad for a triathlete. Remember: Carbohydrates are our primary energy source and are necessary for training and racing, so convert-ing AAs in the body into glucose adds to this energy source. However, on the other hand, those AAs used to make new glucose have to come from somewhere. Since the body cannot store AAs, it will compensate for a lack of carbohydrates by oftentimes breaking down skeletal muscle protein to provide AAs.

The idea of losing skeletal muscle—and muscle mass—so you can make new glucose probably doesn't sound too appealing, so it's important to get the proper amount of carbohydrates in your diet during training and racing. You also do not want to restrict total calories too much if you are trying to lose weight.

I cannot stress this last point enough: As a triathlete, you should never be on a low-carbohydrate diet. These diets may be popular among mainstream Americans, but they have no place in the world of triathlons. You need those carbohydrates, and if you don't provide enough of them for your body, your body will find a way to make them at the expense of skeletal muscle, and your mood. So, ignore the low-carb craze and get adequate amounts of both carbohydrates and protein on a daily basis.

CHAPTER 3

Fats

The phrase dietary fat tends to make people shudder—mostly because they view fat as the enemy. Triathletes are no different. They see it as something that keeps them from their ideal race weight or increases their risk of heart disease.

Well, I'm here to say that fat tends to get a bad rap. Yes, too much fat can definitely lead to weight gain. However, too much of your other macronutrients (carbs and protein) will do the same thing. So don't view fat as the enemy. For triathletes, fat serves as an important energy source; in fact, some fat in your diet is essential. Therefore, don't skip over this chapter, because this macronutrient is important for both your health and your training/racing.

Types of Fat

There are three types of fat that we get from our food:

1. Triglycerides

2. Phospholipids

3. Sterols

The most common are triglycerides. In fact, about 98 percent of the fat we eat is in the form of triglycerides. During digestion your body has to break them down, which generally takes longer to accomplish than it does for some other nutrients (such as carbohydrates). Because of this digestion delay, if you eat fat before you train, you will need to allow plenty of time for digestion and absorption to occur. Having dietary fat in the GI tract when you exercise can cause some GI distress. Because fats take longer to digest and absorb, many triathletes limit fat intake or avoid it altogether right before or during exercise.

Most of the fatty acids in triglycerides are called long-chain fatty acids. This differs from the medium-chain triglycerides (MCTs) that are marketed as ergogenic aids for endurance athletes. The theory behind MCTs is that they can be digested and absorbed much more rapidly than regular long-chain triglycerides, meaning that they provide a more-immediate energy source to the body during low- to moderate-intensity exercise. Most of the research does not support this theory, however, and some people still get GI complications from MCTs, so I do not recommend them. (Save your money for something else. This sport is expensive enough without adding costs for things that don't really work.)

When discussing fatty acids in triglycerides, you have to talk about the degree of saturation. To keep your eyes from glazing over here, I'm going to keep it simple and straightforward. You actually probably already know something about this. Ever heard of trans, saturated, or omega fats? Saturated fatty acids (SFAs) tend to be solid at room temperature and are not heart-healthy. Unsaturated fatty acids—monounsaturated fatty acids (MUFAs), which contain one double bond in the structure—and polyunsaturated fatty acids (PUFAs), which contain more than one double bond in the structure—are healthier fats. Trans fats are the worst fatty acids for you. Very few trans fats exist naturally; rather, most are the result of chemical modifications, where a healthy unsaturated fat is turned into a trans fat. They were first created to preserve the shelf life of products in order to prevent or delay rancidity (spoilage). Of course, now we know about the dangers and harmful effects of these fats.

The second category of lipids is phospholipids. We consume very few phospholipids in our diet and can actually synthesize them in our body, so they are not essential fats. Fat is insoluble in water. Phospholipids are unique because they contain both a fat-soluble component and a water-soluble component. This means that they have the ability to be soluble (or mix well) in water. Their functions in the body are a result of this unique characteristic.

The third category of lipids is sterols. These come from plant sources (plant sterols) or animal sources (cholesterol and others). Plant sterols actually have health benefits. Animal sterols, the primary one being cholesterol, also have some important functions in the body. However, too much cholesterol (or too much of the wrong type of cholesterol) can increase your risk of developing heart disease.

Health Benefits of Fat

I know, I know—you're thinking there can't possibly be any health benefits derived from fat. However, fat and cholesterol have a big impact on your overall health and disease risk. There are actually "good" fats out there that can decrease your risk of developing chronic illnesses such as cardiovascular disease. Unfortunately, there are also "bad" fats that increase the risk of such diseases. Different types of fatty acids have different disease risks associated with them; for example, SFAs and trans fats greatly increase the risk of cardiovascular disease. It's important to focus on getting as many MUFAs and PUFAs for your fat calories as possible; to keep your SFAs to less than 10 percent of your total calories; and to limit your trans-fat intake as much as possible—all of which will lead to a healthier diet and a longer life. Later in this chapter (under "Food Sources of Fat" on page 30) I will provide some examples of foods that contain either "good" or "bad" fats.

MUFAs and PUFAs do not appear to increase your risk for developing chronic disease, and certain types of these fatty acids—omega fats—actually have very important functions in the body. Omega fats (omega-3, omega-6, and omega-9 fatty acids) have received a lot of press in recent years. Omega-3 and omega-6 fatty acids are essential fatty acids, while omega-9 is a nonessential fatty acid. This means that your body cannot synthesize omega-3 or -6 fatty acids, so you must obtain them from your diet. Omega-3 and omega-6 fatty acids are PUFAs with important health implications. Both are important for proper brain function, as well as for normal growth and development.

While both of these omega fatty acids have several important functions in the body, omega-3 fatty acids are especially good for you, as they help to reduce inflammation and clotting, which lowers your risk for cardiovascular disease. Conversely, omega-6 fatty acids actually promote or increase inflammation and blood clotting. Excess omega-6 fatty acids can also interfere with the health benefits of omega-3 fatty acids. Therefore, the ratio of omega-3 to omega-6 fatty acids in the diet is important for reducing the risk of cardiovascular disease; however, the exact ratio needed is still undetermined. The recommended ratio varies from 5:1 to 10:1 omega-6 to omega-3, while others suggest that optimal ratios would be between 1:1 and 4:1. It is estimated that most adults actually eat a ratio of 14:1 to 20:1 of omega-6 to omega-3.

Now, let's talk a little about cholesterol. Again, since I want to keep this as simple as possible, we'll only discuss total cholesterol, high-density lipoprotein (HDL) cholesterol, and low-density lipoprotein (LDL) cholesterol. In general, high amounts of cholesterol will increase your risk for atherosclerosis (or, fat buildup in your arteries) and cardiovascular disease. Your body synthesizes cholesterol, so sometimes the amount of cholesterol in your body cannot be controlled by what you eat. If you are someone who has high cholesterol, then you'll need to take other measures to control the cholesterol amounts, such as decrease your dietary cholesterol intake, increase your fiber intake, and decrease your SFA and trans-fat intake. The recommendation for adults is to eat less than 300mg of total cholesterol per day.

To make things just a little more complicated, you have both good and bad types of cholesterol in the body. HDL cholesterol is your "good" cholesterol. It actually helps prevent fat buildup in your arteries. Conversely, LDL cholesterol is your "bad" cholesterol, because it deposits fat onto the walls of your arteries. If you haven't had your cholesterol checked in a while, it's probably a good idea to do so. Below is a table of desirable, borderline, and high-cholesterol profiles. The great thing for you, the triathlete, is that exercise raises your HDL, or good, cholesterol. This means that you likely have high HDL levels because of your triathlon training.

	DESIRABLE	BORDERLINE HIGH	UNDESIRABLE
Total Cholesterol	<200mg/dL	200–239mg/dL	≥240mg/dL
LDL Cholesterol	<100mg/dL	130–159mg/dL	≥160mg/dL
HDL Cholesterol	≥60mg/dL	40–59mg/dL	<40mg/dL

Functions of Fat in the Body

Despite what most people believe, fats are actually essential for the body to function properly, and they play a bigger role than just being a storage form of energy in the body. A major function of fat is to be an energy source. We use fat for energy at low to moderate intensities of exercise, as well as throughout the day and during sleep. Fats provide more than twice as much energy as either carbohydrates or proteins (9 calories per gram), and, unlike carbs and proteins, your body has the ability to store an almost unlimited amount of fat.

Some of the other functions of fat depend on the type of fat. Triglycerides, for example, not only provide a major energy source, but they also provide protection around vital organs, insulate the body, transport fat-soluble vitamins in the body, induce satiety (feelings of fullness), and provide flavor to food.

Phospholipids make up a very small portion of our diet, but they have important functions because they contain both a water-soluble and a fat-soluble component. Therefore, they often act as emulsifiers and transporters in the body, and they also make up cell membranes. Your body can synthesize phospholipids, so it is not essential to get them in your diet.

Make Note: Fats are a good source of energy for the body, as they provide 9 calories per gram. They are also a primary energy source during low-intensity exercise.

Sterols come from either plant sources (plant sterols) or animal sources (cholesterol and others). Plant sterols can actually help lower LDL (bad) cholesterol, so they are considered heart-healthy. Cholesterol is the most common animal-derived sterol and is something even your healthiest triathletes should limit. Although cholesterol usually gets a pretty bad rap, it is important for the body. Cholesterol is used to create good membrane permeability and fluidity of cells, and it is converted into bile, which is important for digestion and absorption of dietary fats.

Food Sources of Fat

Fat adds a lot of flavor to foods, so just about anything that tastes really good has some fat in it. Fats that are derived from plant sources are generally healthier than fats from animal sources. This means they have more MUFAs and PUFAs and fewer SFAs and trans fats. Your plant sources of fats are usually liquid at room temperature and include most of your oils (olive, canola, corn, vegetable, soybean, flaxseed, cottonseed, coconut oil, and others). Other common plant sources include nuts, seeds, and avocados. Foods rich in omega-3 fatty acids include fish oils and some plant oils (such as flaxseed oil), as well as some nuts (especially walnuts). The omega-6 fatty acids are commonly found in other oils (palm, soybean, rapeseed, and sunflower), as well as nuts, eggs, and avocados. Omega-9 fatty acids are most commonly found in olive oil and canola oil.

Animal sources of fat typically have more SFAs than plant sources. These include those found in dairy products (as long as they are not fat-free, of course), such as cheese, milk, yogurt, ice cream, and butter. Most meats also contain fats—some more than others. Additionally, most sauces and creams are rich in fat; this includes salad dressings, gravy, mayonnaise, etc. Finally, nearly all desserts or baked goods are very rich in fats (and not usually the healthy ones). If you are trying to cut back on the amount of fat in your diet, cut back on desserts, choose low-fat and fat-free items if they are available, and make sure you get some healthy fats in your diet (some oils, nuts, and seeds).

Some foods are rich in all three different kinds of fat (triglycerides, phospholipids, and sterols). Since triglycerides make up 98 percent of the fats we eat in our diet, most of the foods previously mentioned are rich in triglycerides (all of the MUFAs, PUFAs, SFAs, and trans fats). Good sources of phospholipids include egg yolks, soybeans, and peanuts. Plant sterols are found in many vegetable oils, nuts, and seeds, while cholesterol is found primarily in meats, desserts, and egg yolks.

General Intake Recommendations for Adults and Triathletes

The AMDR (acceptable macronutrient distribution range) for fat intake is 20 to 35 percent of total calories from fat, which applies both to adults and to triathletes. You do not want to go below 20 percent, considered a "low-fat" diet, because there are important functions for fat in the body. You also do not want to go above 35 percent, because then you probably are not getting enough of your other macronutrients (carbohydrates or protein). While 35 percent sounds awfully high, you should know that the average fat intake in US adults is about 33 percent of total calories.

Make Note: Triathletes should get 20 to 35 percent of their total calories from fat. The focus should be on healthy, unsaturated fats while minimizing saturated and trans-fat intake.

It is not uncommon to see 25 to 30 percent of calories from fat in many tri-athletes. When you plan out your diet or meals, follow the "fat as filler" guideline. What does this mean? This means that you should figure out your carbohydrate and protein needs and then just fill in the rest of your calories with fat.

If you use the correct recommendations for carbohydrates and protein, then your fat intake will fall within the recommended ranges. For example, if you get 60 percent of your calories from carbohydrates and 15 percent from protein, that leaves 25 percent of your calories to come from fat. If you are trying to lose weight, fat calories are usually the first thing that you can cut, although I don't recommend going lower than 20 percent of total calories on the fat intake. Remember, fat is an important energy source for training.

There are also various suggestions for the different types of fat. For example, additional recommendations include limiting saturated fat to less than 10 percent of your total calories, and keeping your trans-fat intake as low as possible. There is such a huge push to eliminate trans fats that there isn't even a percentage associated with the recommended intake. However, if you can't completely eliminate trans fats, then try to limit the intake to as little as possible. For omega-3 fatty acids, the adequate intake is set at 1.6 grams per day for men and 1.1 grams per day for women. Omega-6 recommendations are 17 grams per day for males and 12 grams per day for females.

When it comes to getting fat in your diet, I think the important things to focus on are getting healthy fats (MUFAs and PUFAs, from food sources like olive oil, nuts, seeds, and avocado) and recognizing that, even as a triathlete, you need fat in your diet for healthy body functioning and energy throughout the day and for training sessions.

CHAPTER 4

Vitamins

N ow that we've covered macronutrients, it's time to move on to micronutrients. Vitamins are essential nutrients (meaning your body needs to get them from your diet), but they do not provide any calories or energy; as a result, they are called micronutrients. Your body also needs vitamins in much smaller quantities than your macronutrients (carbohydrates, protein, fat), which is another reason they are called micronutrients. Despite their "micro" status, these nutrients are important, as they have literally hundreds of functions in the body. Eating a balanced, healthy diet ensures that you will meet all of your vitamin needs.

> **Make Note:** If you are eating a balanced, healthy diet, you will meet all of your micronutrient needs. However, I recommend a daily multivitamin/mineral pill as an insurance policy, in order to meet those needs.

I recommend that people take a daily multivitamin/mineral pill; consider it extra coverage. If you normally eat a healthy diet and use the multivitamin supplement as an insurance policy (for days when you don't), you will be sure all of your vitamin needs are met. That being said, I am generally not a supporter of supplements, particularly megadoses of an individual vitamin. Spending tons of money on B vitamins or antioxidant vitamin supplements is

---

DIETARY RECOMMENDATION TERMS
What is a DRI, RDA, or AI?

The dietary reference intake (DRI) is basically an umbrella term used to describe all of the other terms—such as RDA and AI—that are used for nutrient recommendations. A recommended dietary allowance (RDA) is set so that the RDA of a given nutrient will meet the needs of 98 percent of individuals in a healthy population. This basically means that if you get the RDA of a nutrient, you are most likely meeting your body's need for that nutrient. Sometimes there is not enough research for an RDA to be established. If that is the case, an adequate intake (AI) may be listed. An AI is the amount or level of a nutrient that is commonly eaten in a healthy population of people that are free from disease. This basically means that it is probably an adequate amount of that nutrient for your body to function properly.

---

mostly a waste. Once your body gets its required amount, it will just excrete the extra. This means that if you buy B vitamins, which provide two to four times the recommended amount, you are just making expensive urine. Save your money for something that's actually beneficial to your body.

Vitamins have several different functions, but I am going to focus only on their major functions here. In addition to discussing the major functions of each vitamin, I have included a DRI (dietary reference intake) table in the appendix that lists the RDA (recommended dietary allowance) or AI (adequate intake) for each vitamin, for a number of age groups in both men and women.

Your vitamins can be broken into two different categories: fat-soluble vitamins and water-soluble vitamins. Your fat-soluble vitamins are vitamins A, D, E, and K. Your water-soluble vitamins are vitamins B and C. The fat-soluble vitamins need dietary fat in order to be digested and absorbed (so take your multivitamin with food that contains fat). Since your body can store fat-soluble vitamins, it takes a very long time to see deficiencies, and you can get toxic levels if you take in too much of any one of them. Conversely, the water-soluble vitamins are not readily stored in the body, so any excess gets excreted in urine. This means that you need to consume these on a daily basis; signs and symptoms of deficiencies do not take as long to show up, and toxicity is much rarer. We will not cover toxicity or deficiency of vitamins in this chapter.

B Vitamins and Choline

Functions: You have several B vitamins. They include: B1 (thiamine), B2 (riboflavin), B3 (niacin), B5 (pantothenic acid), B6 (pyridoxal phosphate), B7 (biotin), B9 (folate), and B12 (cobalamin). While your B vitamins are essential for hundreds of reactions and functions in the body, in general, they are very important for energy production. Do not confuse energy production with containing energy. Your B vitamins do not contain energy (this means they do not contain calories). So, eating more B1 will not directly give you more energy because B1 does not have any calories.

Your B vitamins do help to create energy-producing pathways in the body. Your body has several different metabolic pathways that it uses to produce energy from carbs, protein, and fats. The B vitamins have several important roles in those metabolic pathways, and therefore help your body to produce energy for you to use. As you might suspect, the higher your metabolism (i.e., the more carbs, protein, and fat your body burns for energy), the more B vitamins you need. Therefore, triathletes who burn a lot of calories may have a slightly higher need for B vitamins than your average couch potato. Still, that does not mean that you need to take B vitamin supplements. If you eat a healthy diet and take a multivitamin supplement daily, you will get plenty of B vitamins.

Choline is a compound that is listed in this category even though it is not a vitamin. (Your body can synthesize choline, so it's not essential to get it in your diet.) Choline is an important component of acetylcholine, which helps with muscle contraction (it transmits signals from the brain and nerve cells to working muscles). Choline is also important for energy production, which is why it's included in this section.

Food Sources: In general, if you eat a healthy diet, you will meet the nutrient requirements for each of these B vitamins. Some foods rich in certain B vitamins include sweet potato (rich in B1); dairy products (rich in B2); fortified grains (rich in many B vitamins); cereal products (rich in many B vitamins); whole grains (rich in many B vitamins); bran and bran cereals (rich in B6 and B9); meats and seafood such as tuna, turkey, chicken, beef (rich in B3); clams and oysters (rich in B12); spinach and beans (rich in B9 and B7); mushrooms (rich in B5); yogurt (rich in B2 and B5); and egg yolks (rich in choline and B7). This is a very general list; there are many other foods that contain small or large amounts of B vitamins. This list is just a general guide to show you a few items that are rich in certain nutrients, and to also show that most healthy foods—such as whole grains, fruits and vegetables, dairy products, and meats—are good sources of B vitamins and choline.

Vitamin C, Vitamin E, and Vitamin A

Functions: I have grouped these three vitamins together because they have important antioxidant functions in the body. Antioxidants fight free radicals in your body. Free radicals can be introduced into the body through a number of environmental factors, such as tobacco smoke, pollution, medications, radiation, and charred foods. Oxygen, nitrogen, and some minerals (iron and copper) can also cause free-radical damage. Free radicals damage cells in the body, and it is the job of antioxidants to stop this damage. Oxygen is one of the major culprits of free-radical damage in the body; as a result, athletes produce more free radicals because they use more oxygen during exercise.

One cool thing about the human body is its ability to counteract negative things. One of the adaptations to exercise training is that your body's defense systems against free radicals are enhanced. Therefore, even though you produce more free radicals by exercising, your body is much better at fighting them off. Still, it is important for you to make sure you get enough antioxidant vitamins to help fight off free-radical damage. Once again, if you eat a healthy diet, then you will get enough antioxidant vitamins.

You also do not want to take supplements containing large doses of these vitamins (especially vitamin A), because you can get to toxic levels. Therefore, I recommend a healthy diet and a daily multivitamin as an insurance policy but advise against large doses on a frequent basis. These three vitamins also have other functions aside from their role as antioxidants. Vitamin C is important for collagen formation and can enhance the absorption of iron in the body, and vitamin A plays an important role in vision and the immune system.

Food Sources: Food sources for vitamin C include just about anything in the citrus category (oranges, pineapples, strawberries, mango, and cantaloupe), as well as tomato juice, spinach, broccoli, cauliflower, and sweet potato. Vitamins A and E are fat-soluble, so they are found in foods that contain fat. Vitamin E is readily found in several oils (wheat-germ, cottonseed, safflower, and corn), as well as in almonds, hazelnuts, sunflower seeds, and peanuts. Food sources that are rich in vitamin A include liver, sweet potato, carrots, spinach, peppers, broccoli, romaine lettuce, cantaloupe, and oatmeal. There are several other foods that contain these vitamins; these are just a few examples to get you started.

Vitamin D and Vitamin K

Functions: Vitamin D is known as your "sunshine" vitamin because ultraviolet (UV) exposure on the skin stimulates the synthesis of vitamin D in the body. However, much of the vitamin D that your body needs comes from your diet. Vitamin D is important for regulating blood calcium levels and for bone growth, development, and maintenance of bone mineral density. Vitamin K can also be synthesized in the body (in the large intestine by gut bacteria), but the majority of it needs to come from your diet. Vitamin K's primary function is to help the body form blood clots when necessary, but it also has a minor role in bone maintenance.

Food Sources: Cod-liver oil is an exceptional source of vitamin D. Other good sources include canned salmon and sardines, as well as milk. Foods rich in vitamin K include spinach, turnip greens, cauliflower, broccoli, and romaine lettuce.

The functions of the vitamins described here are by no means their only functions. As I mentioned earlier, vitamins are involved in hundreds of reactions in the body. This introduction gives you some highlights of their major functions and how important it is for triathletes to get adequate amounts on a daily basis. Because vitamins play such an important role in the body, many triathletes look to supplement their diets with an individual vitamin or group of vitamins. I will address supplementation in chapter 12, but here's the take-home message on vitamin supplementation: If you have adequate levels of micronutrients, additional supplementation above the recommended amount will not enhance your athletic performance. Supplementing with a vitamin or group of vitamins will only affect exercise performance if you have a deficiency in said vitamin.

CHAPTER 5

Minerals

Minerals are the other category of micronutrients. They are essential, so you must get minerals from your diet, but you do not need them in large amounts. Like vitamins, minerals do not provide any energy (they do not have calories), but they do have a variety of important functions in the body. I will not discuss all of the minerals in this chapter, and I will stick to only one or two main functions of each, despite the fact that most minerals have several functions. You can get your daily recommended amount of each of these minerals by eating a healthy, balanced diet, but I know that not all triathletes do this all of the time. Therefore, I suggest taking a multivitamin pill each day as an insurance policy to make sure you meet your daily needs.

Sodium, Potassium, Chloride, Phosphorus, and Calcium

Functions: The major function of sodium, potassium, and chloride is their role as electrolytes. Calcium and phosphorus are also electrolyte minerals that possess other important/primary functions (to be discussed in later sections).

In general, electrolytes regulate fluid balance, help nerves respond to stimuli, and signal muscles to contract. Sodium, potassium, and chloride are very important for regulating fluid balance in the body and are lost from the body through sweat. This means that the more you sweat, the more electrolytes you lose. This is especially true for sodium, as your sweat contains more sodium than it does potassium or chloride. Since triathletes train so much more than most recreational athletes, having enough electrolytes is quite important. I will discuss electrolyte replacement and usage during training/racing in part two of this book (see page 55).

Make Note: Electrolytes—especially sodium—are lost through sweat. Triathletes who exercise for longer than ninety minutes need to consume electrolytes through foods or sports drinks/products in order to replace what has been lost.

As part of their everyday diet, most triathletes get plenty of sodium, potassium, and chloride. In fact, your sodium intake is usually much higher than the RDA, so you probably don't need to worry about getting more salt in your diet. That is one benefit to working out so much: Unlike most Americans, who have to try to reduce their salt intake, as a triathlete, you don't have to worry as much about that. Some triathletes, however, have high blood pressure. If you are one of them, you probably can't go crazy with your salt intake, but you will be able to consume more than a sedentary individual.

Potassium intake tends to be a little low in the average American's diet. This is mostly due to the fact that potassium is commonly found in fruits and vegetables, and most Americans do not eat enough of those. If you eat a healthy diet, you will get adequate amounts of all three of these electrolytes, and will not need to increase your intake on a daily basis. You should never take potassium tablets, as potassium can cause heart arrhythmias. Just stick to a healthy diet, and you will be fine.

Food Sources: It's quite easy to get sodium and chloride from our food supply. Anything with salt will be rich in both sodium and chloride. In addition to salt, canned or processed foods are usually rich in both sodium and chloride. Other rich sources include soy sauce, condiments, fast food, smoked meats, and soups. Conversely, potassium is primarily found in natural or healthier foods. Foods rich in potassium include potatoes, spinach, bananas, meat, milk, coffee, and tea. Most sports-nutrition products also contain sodium, potassium, and sometimes chloride. This includes most sports drinks, gels, and bars.

Selenium

Function: Selenium is an antioxidant. For a refresher on the function of antioxidants, see page 35. Selenium is the one mineral that has a major function as an antioxidant. In addition to its important antioxidant function, selenium is also used for immune function and thyroid function.

Food Sources: Animal products, especially seafood, are rich in selenium. Good sources include oysters, canned tuna, lobster, pork loin, shrimp, spaghetti, whole-wheat bread, eggs, and oatmeal.

Calcium, Phosphorus, Magnesium, and Fluoride

Functions: Several minerals are important for bone growth, development, and maintenance. Bone maintenance is something all adults—not just growing kids—should be concerned with. Calcium, phosphorus, magnesium, and fluoride have a primary function in maintaining bone mineral density. Calcium, which is the most abundant mineral in your body, has some other important roles in addition to bone formation. It is involved in muscle contraction, nerve transmission, blood clotting, and, in recent years, has been shown to decrease the risk of colon cancer and may lower blood pressure. Phosphorus works in conjunction with calcium to increase bone mineral density, but it also forms cell membranes in the body and is a component of our body's form of chemical energy. Like calcium, magnesium plays a role in blood-clot formation, helps regulate blood pressure, and has some important metabolic functions. Fluoride primarily helps to deposit calcium and phosphorus in bones and teeth, but it also helps to prevent cavities and improves ligament and tendon strength.

Food Sources: Unfortunately, most people do not consume enough calcium. The dietary guidelines suggest three cups a day of low-fat and/or fat-free dairy products. This is because dairy products (yogurt, milk, cheese) are rich sources of calcium. Provolone cheese is also rich in phosphorus, along with yogurt, sunflower seeds, bran cereal, milk, and some meats, such as beef and chicken. Foods that are rich in magnesium include bran cereal, sesame seeds, halibut, almonds, oysters, cashews, and soybeans. Water is the main source of fluoride (bottled water usually has a lower fluoride content), which means that you will get fluoride from most beverages, as well as foods that are prepared in water. Additionally, most toothpastes and mouthwashes contain fluoride.

If you are prone to stress fractures or bone breaks, then you may want to consider calcium and/or vitamin D supplements. However, I suggest consulting with your physician first. For most triathletes, if you focus on meeting the dietary guidelines and you take a multivitamin/mineral as an insurance policy, then you should be able to easily meet your needs for these minerals.

Iron, Zinc, Copper, and Iodine

Functions: The minerals in this category all have several important functions in the body. I feel it is necessary to at least mention one or two main functions for each of them. I will start with iron. Iron is the number-one micronutrient deficiency in the United States. Low iron status is much more common in women than men because of monthly losses of iron during menstruation. Conversely, iron can be toxic at high doses and can also do free-radical damage on the body, so you do not want to take too much.

Iron deficiency is quite prevalent in female athletes. Iron is especially important for triathletes because it is a component of hemoglobin (Hb) and myoglobin, which are essential for transporting and utilizing oxygen. Therefore, if you have low iron, your hemoglobin and red blood cell count may be low, which means you can't transport or utilize as much oxygen as you should. This will have a huge impact on your athletic capabilities. You may also feel fatigue, low energy, and cold intolerance if you do not have enough iron. If you experience any of these symptoms (more so than what is typical for a triathlete), you may want to pay your doctor a visit to get your iron status tested.

Zinc and copper have literally hundreds of functions and assist with several important systems in the body. Zinc, specifically, is important for wound healing and protein synthesis, and it also helps with metabolism (producing energy). Copper assists with iron transport in the body, helps protect against free-radical damage, and assists with metabolism. The last mineral in this section is iodine, which really has just one function in the body—to assist in the synthesis of thyroid hormones. Those hormones play an important role in weight control, energy expenditure, and temperature regulation.

41

Food Sources: One of the reasons that iron deficiency is so prevalent in adult females is because iron is not found in a huge variety of foods, and athletes often avoid or limit their intake of foods that are rich in iron. Beef, or red meat, is an excellent example. It has modest amounts of iron, but many triathletes—females in particular—try to limit their intake of red meat. If you have low iron, then the occasional hamburger or steak may be just what you need. Other good sources of iron include clams, oysters, and some cereals (i.e., All-Bran, Cheerios, and cornflakes). Foods that have modest amounts of iron include lentils, shrimp, spinach, tofu, and lima beans. Since most of you female triathletes do not meet your iron needs, taking a multivitamin/mineral pill daily will help ensure that you are not limiting your athletic abilities.

Foods rich in zinc include most animal products, especially beef and other dark meats, crab, and some plant products (whole grains, wheat germ, and legumes). Oysters happen to be a very rich source of both zinc and copper. Other foods rich in copper include lobster, crab, clams, sunflower seeds, hazelnuts, and mushrooms. Iodine is most commonly found in salt (assuming your label says "Iodized Salt"), as well as cod, milk, white bread, and four tortillas.

Other Important Minerals

There are a number of other minerals that we get in our diet that are needed for optimal health and proper body functioning, including chromium, sulfur, manganese, and molybdenum. Additionally, there are some other minerals that do show up in the food supply but do not have an RDA and do not appear to have any biological function in humans. These include arsenic, boron, nickel, silicon, and vanadium.

Minerals are popular choices for supplementation. If an athlete is deficient in a mineral, then supplementing with that mineral to bring their status back up to normal levels may result in an increase in exercise performance. For example, if anemic athletes take iron supplements, they will likely see an increase in aerobic capacity because they are able to bring their oxygen-carrying capacity up to a normal, healthy level. However, for triathletes who are not deficient in any mineral, taking supplements of any given mineral will not increase their exercise performance. In other words, if you are not deficient in a mineral to begin with, you will not receive additional benefits by supplementing your diet with added amounts of that mineral.

CHAPTER 6

Fluids

As I mentioned in the introduction, the three most important nutritional concerns for triathletes are carbohydrates, sodium, and fluids. Water is an essential nutrient for everyone (55 to 60 percent of our bodies are made up of water); we can live for weeks without food but only for a couple of days without water. For athletes, water and fluid intake is even more crucial. We've all heard about the "eight cups a day" guideline, but is that enough fluid for triathletes? What type and how much fluid should triathletes consume before, during, and after training and races? What happens to performance if dehydration occurs? These are just a few of the important questions that will be addressed in this chapter.

Cardiac Drift

As an exercise physiologist, I learned about cardiac drift a number of years ago. It wasn't until I started monitoring my own heart rate during training that I began to truly understand the importance of that term. By definition, cardiac drift is an increase in heart rate without a change in exercise intensity. Basically, this means that if you run the same pace mile after mile, your heart rate will begin to increase over time rather than stay fairly constant. So what causes this? Cardiac drift occurs as you lose blood volume. How do you lose blood volume? Simply put, by sweating; the more you sweat, the more body fluid you lose, including blood volume (your blood is about 90 percent water). Therefore, if you try to pump out the same amount of blood (and oxygen) to working muscles during exercise but lose blood volume through sweat, your body compensates by increasing its heart rate. Now your body still pumps out the same amount of blood (and oxygen) each minute, but your heart works harder to do it.

Most triathletes are aware of the phrase maximal heart rate. You have a maximum rate at which your heart can beat (a good estimate for this is the formula MaxHR = 220 minus your age). There are other, more-complicated formulas, but let's be honest: Sports nutrition is complicated enough, so we'll keep it simple here. Generally, when you exercise, you want your heart rate to be as low as possible. In fact, this is a good way to measure your fitness level. If you perform the same workout each week and monitor your heart rate during that workout, as your fitness improves, your heart rate should go down. Many coaching plans utilize heart rate to measure training intensity.

From a sports-nutrition perspective, you want to make sure that any changes in your heart rate during a workout come from changes in exercise intensity—not because of dehydration. Now, a small amount of cardiac drift may not seem like that big of a deal. So what if your heart rate goes up 5 bpm (beats per minute) over the course of a one- or two-hour workout? Well, if 5 bpm were all we were talking about, it probably wouldn't be that big of a deal for most triathletes. However, the cardiac drift that can occur during even a one-hour workout can be really severe.

In my own training (on moderately hot, humid days), I've seen my heart rate go up more than 20 bpm in the final twenty or so minutes of an 8- to 10-mile run. This occurs with no change in my running pace. Ask any elite athlete how an increase in heart rate of 20 bpm affects his performance and his answer will undoubtedly be "A lot!" You may go from 70 percent of your maximum up to 85 percent or more without having increased intensity at all. From a performance standpoint, this is just about the worst thing that can happen.

Don't worry—this isn't all bad news. You can try to combat cardiac drift during exercise by consuming fluids while you work out. If you can replace fluids as you lose them through sweat, you can try to prevent a large decrease in blood volume, which means that your heart rate won't have to increase to maintain the same output at a given intensity. The point of all of this is to say that consuming fluids during exercise is crucial—and that's an understatement. Unfortunately, for those who sweat a lot, it is almost impossible to replace all the fluids that will be lost during exercise, but even if you're only able to replace 50 percent of them, that will at least slow down (or delay) cardiac drift.

Dehydration has other detrimental effects on performance, aside from cardiac drift. A major one is muscle cramps. This can occur from dehydration, electrolyte loss, or both. Regardless of the exact cause, muscle cramps will affect your performance (and may make your race day quite painful). If you are prone to muscle cramping, it is especially important for you to ensure adequate fluid intake and to take electrolytes with that fluid.

Sweat Rates

Triathletes all have different sweat rates. This means that two people doing the same exercise in the same conditions will not lose fluid at the same rate. I'm sure you've noticed this if you train with other people. You have your "sweaters" and your "non-sweaters." If you're more of a non-sweater, good for you; it will be easier for you to try to remain hydrated while you train. If you are a sweater, well, then, this chapter is really important for you. You can't do much to change your sweat rate (although it will change some as your fitness improves), so we'll focus on how to deal with the sweat rate you have.

I used to think it was a disadvantage to be a "non-sweater." I played basketball in high school and never sweated too much. I couldn't understand it because I was working just as hard as my teammates, and they looked like they had just walked through a car wash. Back then, I equated sweating with hard work (I think many people still do). I now realize the advantages to being a non-sweater. In terms of maintaining hydration during exercise, I have a huge advantage over my husband (a sweater), simply because I don't lose as many fluids as he does.

Make Note: Every triathlete should calculate their own sweat rate. Since sweat rates will likely vary from one activity to another, sweat trials should be performed for swimming, biking, and running. You want to perform these trials in similar environmental conditions to what you expect to see on race day.

There are a number of factors that can affect your sweat rate during exercise, including environmental conditions (temperature, humidity, and even wind), elevation, size of the individual, fitness level, and genetics. Since people sweat at different rates, it is difficult to make recommendations for fluid intake during exercise. I make some general recommendations for fluid intake in this chapter, but if you really want to be accurate, you need to perform a sweat trial. Since your sweat rate will likely vary from one activity to another, you should perform sweat trials for swimming, biking, and running. Ideally, you'll want to perform these in conditions similar to what you will see on race day. As you can imagine, sweat rates will differ greatly in the middle of a Wisconsin winter versus a summer race in Houston, Texas.

Here are the steps for performing your sweat trial:

1. Record your body weight in pounds before and after exercise. If your clothes are really wet with sweat after exercise (or from being in the water), change into similar dry clothes.

2. For each pound of weight lost (sorry—you lost water weight, not pounds of fat), you need 2 to 3 cups of fluid (16 to 24 ounces, with 1 cup equaling 8 ounces), so multiply the pounds of weight lost by 2 and 3 cups.

3. Add in any fluids you consumed during the workout (you will need to keep track of this during the sweat trial).

4. This number is your sweat rate. If you exercised for two hours, divide your number by two to get your sweat rate per hour.

Make sure you don't go to the bathroom during the sweat trial; otherwise, you'll have to try to account for that fluid loss too. By calculating your sweat rate, you can determine the amount of fluid you need to consume per hour to maintain blood plasma levels and prevent dehydration. In the example in the sidebar on page 47, the individual's sweat rate is 3 to 4 cups per hour (24 to 32 ounces per hour). Therefore, to prevent dehydration, this athlete needs to consume 3 to 4 cups (24 to 32 ounces) of fluid per hour.

For those who don't sweat a great deal, it may be easy to consume enough fluids to match losses. However, people who sweat a lot are unlikely to consume fluids at a rate that will match their losses. Most triathletes can

CALCULATING SWEAT RATE:
An Example (in both cups and ounces)

1. Body weight before: 165 pounds. Body weight after: 163 pounds. Total weight loss: 2 pounds.
2. 2 pounds lost x 2 to 3 cups of fluid per pound = 4 to 6 cups (32 to 48 ounces).
3. Consumed 2 cups (16 ounces) of fluid during workout, so 4 to 6 cups + 2 cups = 6 to 8 cups (32 to 48 ounces + 16 ounces = 48 to 64 ounces).
4. Exercised for two hours, so 6 to 8 cups divided by 2 = 3 to 4 cups per hour (48 to 64 ounces divided by 2 = 24 to 32 ounces per hour).

only absorb about 4 cups of fluid per hour on the bike, and about 2 to 3 cups of fluid per hour on the run. Therefore, if your sweat rate is 6 cups per hour on the bike or run, you probably will not be able to match fluid intake with loss. It is still important to perform sweat trials so you know how much fluid you lose per hour, and to try to minimize those losses by taking in as much as possible.

Rehydration

Even if you perform sweat trials to calculate fluid needs and try to match intake with your sweat losses, you will likely still be slightly dehydrated when you finish exercising. Many triathletes exercise on a daily basis and often perform multiple workouts within the same day. Therefore, recovery after workouts becomes a very important issue. If you are slightly dehydrated from a morning bike ride and do not rehydrate properly, your afternoon run is likely going to be subpar. Weigh yourself before and after your training session. For every pound of weight lost, you need to drink 2 to 3 cups (16 to 24 ounces) of fluid to adequately rehydrate. Begin rehydrating right after exercise and continue to drink those fluids until you have consumed the correct amount (calculated based on weight loss from the training session). If you don't have access to a bathroom scale, then continue to drink fluids until your urine is a pale yellow color, and/or you urinate about once every one to two hours.

> **Make Note:** For every pound of weight lost during exercise, you need to drink 2 to 3 cups (16 to 24 ounces) of fluid to adequately rehydrate. If you don't have access to a scale, drink fluids until your urine is a pale yellow color.

Fluid Recommendations

There are a couple of different recommendations that you can follow for general daily fluid consumption. The table on the following page includes daily fluid consumption recommendations for the average adult, based on the DRI (daily recommended intake). Note that this table does not take into account water lost through sweating. We will discuss that next. For your reference, the table is in liters (L). There are 4.2 cups per liter.[2] Therefore, you will need to multiply the values in the table by 4.2 if you want to see your recommended water intake in cups per day.

Approximately 20 to 25 percent of the water that you consume will come from foods, but the majority of it comes from beverages. This daily fluid consumption recommendation is just the starting point for triathletes; it does not take into account fluids lost during training. Therefore, while this table is useful, there are different intake recommendations for triathletes. The drawback of the triathlete recommendation is that you have to know approximately how many calories you burn each day, because your fluid intake recommendation is based on energy expenditure. If you eat about 2,500 calories a day and you are not changing body weight, then your energy expenditure is about 2,500 calories a day.

The triathlete intake recommendation actually has two parts to it:

1. The recommended water intake is 1 milliliter of water for every calorie expended. So, if you burn 2,500 calories a day, then you need 2,500 milliliters (or 2.5 liters) of water each day. Remember

---

2   AI = Adequate intake in liters per day. There are 4.2 cups per liter.

to multiple each liter by 4.2 to get cups (2.5 liters x 4.2 cups per liter = 10.5 cups).

2. Then, add the amount of water lost during exercise (i.e., sweat loss). To calculate this, you need pre- and post-exercise body weights. For every pound lost during the training session, you need to drink 2 to 3 cups of water. If you lost 2 pounds during exercise, then you need an additional 4 to 6 cups (2 x 2 to 3 cups) of water.

DAILY FLUID CONSUMPTION BY GENDER AND AGE GROUP

	MALES				FEMALES			
	4–8 yrs.	9–13 yrs.	14–18 yrs.	>19 yrs.	4–8 yrs.	9–13 yrs.	14–18 yrs.	>19 yrs.
From Foods	0.5	0.6	0.7	0.7	0.5	0.5	0.5	0.5
From Beverages	1.2	1.8	2.6	3.0	1.2	1.6	1.8	2.2
Total Water	1.7	2.4	3.3	3.7	1.7	2.1	2.3	2.7

Source: Information for this table obtained from DRI reports (nap.edu), Institute of Medicine of the National Academies.

Therefore, in our example, your total fluid intake for the day should be 14.5 to 16.5 cups. If you do not want to go through the math to figure out your own specific fluid recommendation, you can follow the table presented here and then add in additional fluid for exercise (2 to 3 cups for each pound lost). Remember also that about 20 to 25 percent of this fluid intake will come from food.

Recommendations for fluid intake before, during, and after both training sessions and races are discussed in detail in part two.

Types of Fluids

Let's talk a little about the beverages that you drink throughout the day and with your meals. These include water, soft drinks, coffee, tea, sports drinks, juice, milk, and alcohol. I may have missed a few, but chances are this list makes up the majority of your fluid intake on a daily basis.

Water is the best fluid choice and should make up at least 75 percent of your daily fluid intake (training sessions aside). Water has many important functions in the body, and it does not have any added calories. This is key, as most triathletes are concerned about their weight. When I coach athletes who want to lose weight, I tell them that the first thing to cut out of their diet is liquid calories. Since water doesn't have any calories, drink away.

There are several different sports drinks on the market today (see the list of the most common sports drinks and their nutritional content in the appendix, page 188). Sports drinks are important for endurance exercise, but, for the most part, there is no real reason why you need to consume sports drinks outside of training. The positive is that sports drinks typically have fewer calories than juice or regular soda, so if you don't want water, this may be a good second or third choice for fluid intake.

Milk is very healthy, providing calcium and vitamin D, and should be included as part of your daily diet. I recommend low-fat (1 percent) or fat-free milk to reduce the amount of calories and fat. Chocolate milk has more sugar than regular milk (and therefore more calories), so unless you're using it as a recovery drink (which I highly recommend) or trying to gain weight, you should probably only drink this for an occasional treat.

Juice seems to be a popular breakfast drink and can provide some healthy nutrients (some vitamins in particular). However, juice also has a high-sugar content and usually a high-calorie content. Some juices don't even contain any actual fruit juice, so in certain cases you could be drinking sugar water. If you want juice, look for products that contain 100 percent fruit juice so you know you're getting some micronutrients from the product.

Alcoholic beverages . . . I have your attention now, don't I? I know many of you have probably heard that drinking a beer after training or racing is a great recovery aid. Sorry to burst your bubble, but alcoholic beverages are not a good choice for recovery after exercise. If you consume alcohol, it should be in moderation. While wine has been shown to reduce risk of heart disease, in general you won't improve your health much by consuming a lot of alcohol. Furthermore, for the weight-conscious triathlete, alcohol can add a lot of extra calories; in fact, nearly all of the energy from alcohol ends up being stored as fat (some call alcohol "liquid fat" for just this reason).

Alcohol is also a diuretic, meaning it will lead to water loss from the body, so it can cause dehydration if you consume too much and/or do not drink water with it as well. If you enjoy an occasional beer or glass of wine, it will not have much of an effect on your training and performance. However, if you drink quite a bit, it can be detrimental to training and racing and can add on some extra pounds.

Last, but not least, let's discuss those caffeinated beverages. This includes coffee (and all the variations of it), tea, soft drinks, and energy drinks. About 90 percent of the adult population in the United States consumes caffeine on a daily basis, so this section probably applies to you. Caffeine is a drug, which means that you can become addicted to it, but it is fairly safe as long as you consume it in moderation. Caffeine is a stimulant, so it "stimulates" the central nervous system. The end result is increased awareness and alertness.

Like alcohol, caffeine is also a diuretic. In general, you don't want to aim for water loss. Fear not, however; it's not as bad as it sounds. The diuretic effect of caffeine is not a one-to-one ratio, meaning you do not lose 1 cup of fluid for every cup of coffee you drink. It all depends on the caffeine content of the beverage. You will lose about 1 milliliter of fluid for every 1 milligram of caffeine. Therefore, if you drink one 8-ounce cup of coffee (240 milliliters) that contains 80 milligrams of caffeine, you will still have a net fluid gain (240 milliliters gained, 80 milliliters lost).

Where people run into problems is when they consume high amounts of caffeine without a lot of fluid with it (energy drinks, shots of espresso), which can cause dehydration. If you drink caffeine on a daily basis, it is fine to continue to do so as long as it is in moderation and you drink plenty of other fluids with it. You should avoid beverages that have huge amounts of caffeine (such as most energy drinks) because they will not only cause dehydration, but they can also cause some serious heart problems, shakiness, weakness, and difficulty sleeping. The table on the following page lists several popular beverages with their caffeine content.

You must also be careful with the calories from caffeinated beverages. Soft drinks are nearly all sugar, so they are full of empty calories (meaning they lack good nutrients and will not help you feel full). If you love soft drinks, as I do, then at least stick to diet soft drinks. Yes, the acid is terrible for your teeth (and probably your GI tract, too), but at least you won't be expanding your waistline at the same time. The same applies for about half

COMMON BEVERAGES AND FOODS CONTAINING CAFFEINE

PRODUCT	AMOUNT OF CAFFEINE (IN MILLIGRAMS) FOR AN 8-OUNCE (1 CUP) SERVING	PRODUCT SERVING SIZE (IN OUNCES)	CAFFEINE (IN MILLIGRAMS) PER PRODUCT SERVING SIZE
5-hour ENERGY	572	1.93	138
7-Up	0	12	0
AriZona Iced Tea, Green	9	16	15
Coca-Cola Classic	23	12	35
Crystal Light Iced Tea	11	8	11
Diet Coke	30	12	45
Dr Pepper	27	12	41
Canada Dry Ginger Ale	0	12	0
Hershey's Milk Chocolate Bar	62	1.55	12
Hershey's Special Dark Chocolate Bar	138	1.45	25
Lipton Brisk Lemon	7	12	10
McDonald's Small Premium Roast McCafe	73	12	109
Monster Energy	80	16	160
Reese's Peanut Butter Cups	28	1.45	5
Red Bull	76	8.4	80
Shock Coffee Triple Mocha	231	8	231
Snapple Tea	21	16	42
Starbucks Short Coffee	180	8	180
Tazo Chai Tea Latte	47	8	47

of the drinks you can buy at a coffee shop. Plain ol' coffee doesn't have any calories, but some of those fancy lattes and mochas are full of sugar and fat.

Electrolytes and Hyponatremia

You will lose electrolytes (primarily sodium) in your sweat. Actual electrolyte loss is highly variable because it depends on the person's sweat rate; in addition, the amount of electrolytes in that sweat varies from person to person. Therefore, it is impossible to make one recommendation for electrolyte replacement. Electrolyte recommendations are discussed in part two.

Instead, let's discuss hyponatremia, which actually means low blood sodium. This can occur in athletes if they dilute their sodium concentrations in the blood too much. When you sweat, you lose both water and electrolytes. If you only replenish with water, you will begin to dilute electrolyte levels in the blood. Since you lose so much more sodium than any other electrolyte, blood sodium levels can drop severely, leading to hyponatremia. Hyponatremia is very serious, as symptoms can range from nausea, headache, confusion, and fatigue, to muscle cramps, seizures, and decreased consciousness or coma. If severe enough, death can result. To prevent hyponatremia from occurring, make sure that you replace sweat loss with both fluids and electrolytes.

Fluids are important for overall health and are needed in large quantities on a daily basis. For you, the triathlete, fluids are also a necessary part of your training and race-day diet. As we continue to discuss fluids and electrolyte intake throughout this book, refer back to this chapter for the information on sweat rate, diuretic effect of certain drinks, and daily fluid requirements.

Part Two:
The Triathlete's Training and Race-Day Nutrition

Now that you've got the basics down from part one of this book, it's time to get into training and racing nutrition. This is really where all the fun begins. It's important to remember what you've learned from the previous chapters, though, because that knowledge will help you when you're devising your nutrition plans.

One of the great things about the sport of triathlon is that there are so many different racing distances to choose from. On the other hand, this can also complicate things. What you will discover in this section of the book is that some of the nutrition recommendations are the same across the board. This means that whether you're training for a Sprint or full Ironman, a few things will stay the same.

However, most of the recommendations will be specific to the race distance you're aiming for (and of course, the corresponding training volume for that race distance). That is why I have written different chapters for different race distances and included sample meal plans and race-day/training nutrition plans for those different distances (in the appendix). Since you should never do anything new on race day that you haven't already tried during training, let's begin with nutrition during training.

CHAPTER 7

Nutrient Intake Before, During, and After Training Sessions

Nutrition can really affect triathlon performance.

I have done a few triathlons with my friend, Sam, who is a much faster cyclist and runner than I am (although we're about equal in the swim). As expected, he has finished ahead of me in a couple of Sprint triathlons. However, Sam doesn't have very good sports nutrition—we're working on improving it, one step at a time—so when we both competed in the same half Ironman and full Ironman race, guess what happened? Yup—I kicked his butt. As I ran past him both times, all I could think about is how much better he would do if he would just listen to my nutrition advice.

I asked him after the half Ironman race what he had consumed during the race. The answer? About 2 to 3 cups of water and about 200 calories (about 50 grams of carbohydrates). I, on the other hand, had consumed that amount in the first hour of the race alone. The fact that Sam ran out of gas and experienced muscle cramps in the race is proof that sports nutrition can make or break your race, and your training.

In part one you learned what you should be eating on a daily basis. Now we are going to switch gears and talk about nutrition that is specific to your triathlon training. This chapter contains all the nuts and bolts of nutrition for before, during, and after your training sessions. There is quite a large amount of material in this chapter, so take your time reading through it. After you finish this chapter, you should come up with your own nutrition plan for before, during, and after each training session, for one week of training. This may take a little time at first, but most triathletes follow a similar training schedule each week. So, if you can figure out your nutrition plan for one week of training, then you will just need to make minor modifications from week to week after that.

The most important nutrition considerations for triathletes are carbohydrates, fluids, and electrolytes (sodium, in particular). Dehydration will have the most detrimental effect on performance, followed closely by a lack of carbohydrates and not enough electrolytes. Therefore, when nutrition during training sessions is discussed, those three areas always need to be at the forefront.

This chapter is dedicated to aerobic training sessions (swimming, biking, and running); however, there will be some mention of strength training or weight lifting with regard to protein intake. There is a large amount of information, so don't try to absorb it all at once; just take it one step at a time. Start by making small changes to your diet and training sessions, gradually implementing the nutrition advice from this chapter. To help you make the best food decisions for before, during, and after your training sessions, I have included sample meal plans or snack ideas in the appendix.

Training sessions for triathletes are different from training for most other sports because the sessions can be so varied. You may have a short twenty-minute swim on one day and a five-hour bike ride the next. Many triathletes also do multiple workouts in the same day. These workouts may be back to back (which then becomes one long training session), or they may be split up into a morning workout and an afternoon workout. For the latter, you must be sure to get adequate nutrients for the training sessions, as well as for the recovery time in between training sessions. Improper nutrition following that first workout will surely lead to a difficult second workout later in the day.

Since all of these factors need to be considered, nutrition plans for triathletes are also unlike those for athletes in most other sports. As a triathlete, you need to have a nutrition plan for every type of workout—long, short, hard, easy—and for each discipline (swimming, biking, and running). Let's begin by discussing what you should eat right before a training session.

Pre-Training Nutrition

Many triathletes do one of their training sessions first thing in the morning. It's a great way to start your day—as long as you have some breakfast before you get started. Our bodies expend energy during the night, so when you wake up in the morning, your liver is virtually depleted of glycogen. Remember from chapter 1 that glycogen is the storage form of carbohydrate (glucose) in the body; your body relies on that glycogen when you start to exercise. Therefore, you should never start training immediately after an overnight fast. It would be similar to getting into your car when the gas tank is almost empty and trying to coast to work on fumes. Why train on fumes? Carbohydrates and fluids are the most important considerations before a training session, so we will discuss those first.

Carbohydrates: Since carbohydrates are the primary energy source for your body, it is especially important to eat carbohydrates before a training session. The exact amount of carbohydrates varies depending on how many hours before exercise you eat, how much fat and protein are in that meal (as fat and protein will slow down digestion and absorption), and what you are used to eating before exercise. In general, the broad recommendation is 1 to 3.5 grams of carbohydrates per kilogram of body weight any time between one and four hours before exercise. Obviously, if you eat four hours before training, then you may be able to be at the higher end of that recommendation, whereas if you eat one hour before exercise, then the carbohydrate content should be small. The upper end of this recommendation can be a lot of food. Most triathletes never go above 3.5 grams of carbohydrates per kilogram of body weight because it is a lot of food to digest and absorb before a workout (even four hours later). As long as you get more than 1 gram per kilogram, don't worry too much about getting to that upper end of the recommendation.

So here's how you calculate the amount of carbohydrates (and calories) from this recommendation:

Body weight = _____ kilograms

Low end of recommendation:

1. Your weight (in kilograms) x 1 gram per kilogram = _____ grams

2. So, if there are 4 calories per gram of carbohydrate, then
_____ grams x 4 calories per gram = _____ calories

High end of recommendation:

1. _____ kilograms x 3.5 grams per kilogram = _____ grams

2. _____ grams x 4 calories per gram = _____ calories

CALCULATING PRE-TRAINING CARBOHYDRATE INTAKE:
An Example

70-kilogram person (154 pounds)

Low end of recommendation:

1. 70 kilograms x 1 gram per kilogram = 70 grams.
2. So, if there are 4 calories per gram of carbohydrate, then 70 grams x 4 calories per gram = 280 calories.

High end of recommendation:

1. 70 kilograms x 3.5 grams per kilogram = 245 grams.
2. 245 grams x 4 calories per gram = 980 calories.

Let's look at the example calculation. Now, 980 calories just from carbohydrates is quite a significant amount of food to consume before exercising. Again, the high end of this recommendation should only be used if you're three to four hours from exercising (and you are used to eating a large meal before working out). In general, a meal of this size is tolerated better before cycling and swimming, and not as well for running. Therefore, the amount of carbohydrates you eat before a training session may differ depending on what discipline you do. Most athletes eat about two to three hours before exercise. If you eat two to three hours prior to a run workout, I would recommend staying between 1 to 2 grams of carbohydrates per kilogram of body weight. Conversely, if you go for a bike ride or a swim, then eating 2 to 3 grams of carbohydrates per kilogram of body weight, two to three hours prior, should be well tolerated.

One final recommendation on carbohydrate intake: If you eat less than two hours before exercise, there should be minimal amounts of fat and protein in the food; liquid calories are a good option. This will ensure that you can digest and absorb the carbohydrates before you start exercising.

Now that we've discussed the quantity of carbohydrates before exercise, the next question is, what type of carbohydrate? Before exercise, and throughout the rest of the day, low- to moderate-glycemic-index foods are best. Research has shown that eating higher-glycemic-index foods (high-sugar foods) thirty to forty-five minutes before exercise is actually detrimental to exercise performance. Those foods quickly raise blood glucose levels, which leads to a large insulin response. The job of insulin is to clear glucose from the blood, so it promotes the uptake and storage of carbohydrates into tissues. Therefore, when insulin is released after a rapid increase in blood glucose, that glucose is cleared quite rapidly, and blood glucose levels can actually be low at the beginning of exercise. This is the opposite of what you want; during exercise, you want to have plenty of glucose in the bloodstream, and you want the tissues to release those stored carbohydrates so they can all be used for energy. Some people are very sensitive to this, and can actually feel like they are experiencing hypoglycemia if they eat shortly before exercise. Those symptoms (weakness, shakiness, fatigue) will usually go away if you consume some high-sugar foods and stop exercise.

Fluids: You never want to start a training session or competition in a dehydrated state. Unlike carbohydrates, though, you cannot hyperhydrate (overhydrate) and store extra fluid to use during exercise. Taking in a lot of fluids before exercise can lead to cramping and GI distress, frequent urination, and dilution of electrolytes in the blood, if you're consuming only water (see explanation of hyponatremia on page 53). If you don't train right after you get up, fluid considerations for a couple hours before exercise are warranted. You should drink 1 to 2 cups of fluid two hours before exercise, and then drink another cup ten to twenty minutes before you exercise.

Water is a good choice because you don't want to drink anything containing a lot of sugar right before you exercise (as described above). I don't recommend consuming carbonated beverages for up to two hours before exercise; keep in mind that fruit juices tend to have higher carbohydrate concentrations, and milk or dairy products can cause some GI distress. Caffeine can have some performance-enhancing effects (ergogenic properties), but it has diuretic properties as well. If you are used to having some caffeine before exercise, then continue to do so; just keep in mind that it's important to drink water, too, to counteract the diuretic effects of caffeine.

You may not have much spare time to get a lot of fluids in, particularly with morning workouts where, if you're like me, you basically roll out of bed and onto the bike. If this is the case, drink 1 to 2 cups of fluid immediately upon waking to provide at least some initial rehydration from your eight-hour fast during sleep.

Protein: There is very little research on the benefits (or lack thereof) of eating some protein before exercise. While taking in protein before exercise does not seem to enhance aerobic training sessions (swimming, biking, or running), it doesn't seem to have any detrimental effects either. Therefore, if you eat some carbohydrate-rich foods that happen to contain some protein, you shouldn't have anything to worry about.

If your triathlete training also contains strength-training or weight-lifting sessions, then protein intake before exercise does become important. A whole host of studies have proved that taking in protein before a weight-training session has beneficial effects on strength and muscle-mass gains. It helps to prevent protein breakdown in muscle and enhances protein synthesis in muscle after the session. The type of protein consumed before a training session should be complete proteins (which contain all essential amino acids). Remember from chapter 2 that all animal products and soy products contain all nine essential amino acids. The amount of protein needed is also small; as little as 6 to 20 grams of essential amino acids will get the job done.

Fat: Despite the fact that dietary fats make our food taste very good, they are not a welcome friend when it comes to training sessions. My husband can verify that one. As a smart high school student, he decided one day at a track meet that eating a hot dog and nachos before running his 800-meter race was a good idea. He finished the race and continued running—right to the dumpster, where he relieved himself of his "pre-race meal." Enough said.

Dietary fats will slow down or delay digestion and absorption of other nutrients, and they also take a while to digest and absorb themselves. Having a large amount of fat in the GI tract (or any food, for that matter) can lead to GI distress (gas, bloating, cramping, diarrhea) when you start exercising.

Because of this, I recommend you keep fats to a minimum in the four hours prior to exercise. Tolerance to fat tends to vary from person to person, so if you are able to handle some in the hours before exercising, then it won't hurt to have a little. If you will consume a small amount of fat before a training session, try to make it a healthy fat (mono- or polyunsaturated fat) and avoid saturated or trans fats.

Vitamins and Minerals: If you take in adequate amounts of vitamins and minerals on a daily basis, there is no need to consume any extra vitamins or minerals before exercise. Of course, during exercise, you need to think about electrolytes, but you don't have to worry about this before you start.

During-Training Nutrition

For training sessions lasting up to sixty minutes, you do not need carbohydrates or electrolytes, but you should take in fluids. Water is a great choice in this instance. For training sessions lasting longer than sixty minutes, you should take in carbohydrates, electrolytes, and fluids. Here are the specific recommendations for those training sessions lasting longer than sixty minutes.

Carbohydrates: A significant amount of glycogen can be used up during one hour of exercise, so if you exercise for longer than sixty minutes, you should take in carbohydrates. During exercise, you want to supply your body with carbohydrates as quickly as possible. Therefore, I recommend high-glycemic-index foods during exercise because you can digest and absorb them quickly. This means eating and drinking things that have a lot of simple sugars. It is no surprise that most sports drinks, gels, and other food products marketed for exercise contain large amounts of sugar. It is exactly what your body needs.

Make Note: The ideal amount of carbohydrates to consume during exercise is 60 to 70 grams per hour. However, if you are lucky enough to be able to tolerate up to 90 grams per hour, then aim for 90 grams.

As for the amount of carbohydrates to consume, the ideal amount is 60 to 70 grams per hour. There are some individual differences in the amount of carbs that a person can tolerate. Some people can only consume about 45 grams per hour, while others can consume 90 grams per hour. The good thing is that you can train your body to be more tolerant of taking in carbohydrates during training sessions.

My husband is a perfect example of this. When he first started eating gels during training, his stomach would cramp up and he would have to stop consuming the gels; sometimes he would even have to stop exercising altogether if his stomach cramping got severe enough. However, over time he was able to train his body to become accustomed to eating carbohydrates. Keep practicing with the amount you can handle without complications, and then just try adding small amounts to that over a period of time (i.e., an additional 5 grams an hour). Eventually, your body should be able to handle this higher amount. Triathletes can also typically handle food and fluids better on the bike as opposed to during the run. So, if you're trying to train your body to tolerate more carbohydrates, start with implementing more carbs on the bike first before graduating to trying it on the run.

Consuming 60 to 70 grams of carbohydrates per hour is equivalent to 240 to 280 calories. This amount of carbohydrates should be consumed periodically throughout each hour of exercise, and should begin shortly after the onset of exercise. For example, if you do a three-hour bike ride, then you should eat 60 to 70 grams of carbohydrates during each of those three hours. Most gels have about 25 grams of carbohydrate, and 1 cup of a sports drink usually has about 14 grams. Therefore, you can get 60 to 70 grams each hour by eating two gels and 1 to 2 cups of a sports drink. This will help you with your fluid needs as well.

Now, if you don't happen to like gels, you can always try Jelly Belly Sport Beans, Clif Shot Bloks, or any of the other new products on the market that are easy to consume and contain mostly carbohydrates. If you are biking, it is easier to eat solid foods (power bars, crackers, jelly sandwiches, etc.); this is much more difficult to do during swimming and running. The appendix (see page 171) lists some ideas for things to eat and drink during training sessions that will give you the appropriate amount of carbohydrates.

More-recent research shows that the optimal amount of carbohydrates for athletes training for three or more hours is up to 90 grams per hour. Many triathletes cannot handle this much, but if you currently consume 60 to 70 grams per hour, then try adding a few more grams per hour and see how you handle it. You may be able to work your way up to 90 grams per hour.

Finally, the type of carbohydrate is also important. The most easily digested and absorbed carbohydrates are glucose, sucrose, or glucose polymers. High concentrations of fructose have been known to cause GI distress, and they should never be consumed without equal or greater amounts of glucose.

Fluids: The purpose of consuming fluids during training sessions is to maintain both hydration status and electrolyte levels. As I discussed in chapter 6, everyone has his or her own individual sweat rate. I can go out for a training session with some friends and sweat very little, while some of my friends are dripping in sweat after the ten-minute warm-up. Therefore, it is really important for triathletes to perform sweat trials during all facets of training. This means that you need to do a sweat trial for swimming, one for biking, and one for running. The sweat trials also need to be done in weather conditions that are similar to those in which you typically train and/or race. If you perform a sweat trial during the winter when it's 30 degrees Fahrenheit outside, yet you race in July during 80-degree weather, your sweat rate will be very different. If this sounds familiar, it's because I went over all of this in chapter 6. You might want to revisit that chapter again and calculate your sweat rates.

> **Make Note:** If you haven't performed a sweat trial, drink 1 cup of fluid for every ten to twenty minutes of exercise.

If you don't want to calculate a sweat rate, here are general fluid recommendations during exercise. You should drink 1 cup of fluid every ten to twenty minutes of exercise. This should begin soon after the onset of exercise and continue until your training session is complete. Thirst is not a good guide, because your thirst response is delayed. That means, by the time you feel thirsty, you are already partially dehydrated.

Unfortunately, some triathletes sweat profusely and simply cannot match fluid intake with loss. In general, triathletes can only digest and absorb about 1 liter (1,000 milliliters) of fluid per hour on the bike (about 4 cups), and about 500 to 700 milliliters while running (about 2 to 3 cups). So, if your sweat rate is greater than these amounts, you will just have to take in as much fluid as you can handle and recognize that you will slowly dehydrate through the course of your training session.

I often get asked whether sports drinks or water are better to consume during exercise. As a general rule of thumb, if you exercise for less than ninety minutes, you will probably be fine with water alone. However, if you lose a lot of salt in your sweat (you see this salt form on your skin and clothes), or if you exercise in a hot and humid environment, you may need electrolyte replacement for anything over sixty minutes.

Make Note: Consume food or fluids that contain electrolytes, especially sodium, for any exercise lasting longer than ninety minutes.

Any exercise lasting longing than ninety minutes should include electrolytes with the fluids to replace those lost in sweat. This is most easily accomplished with a sports beverage (pick the brand you like best), but can be accomplished with water and solid foods that contain electrolytes. Most triathletes actually see the best results by doing a combination of water and a sports beverage (along with some food to get enough carbohydrates). If it is too difficult to digest and absorb solid foods when exercising at a high intensity, then use a sports beverage that contains the fluids, electrolytes, and carbohydrates you need. Just be careful not to get too many calories or carbohydrates, since some specialty drinks can be pretty nutrient-dense.

There are a lot of different sports drinks available on the market today. Some companies even allow you to design your own drink based on your specifications, and these drinks may provide enough carbohydrate so that no solid foods are needed. I provided a table in the appendix of popular sports drinks, along with their nutritional content (see page 188). Research shows that the best concentration of carbohydrates in a sports drink is a 6 to 8 percent solution. Greater than 8 percent solutions will increase ingestion of carbohydrates, but may delay absorption, and in some instances can even cause bloating, cramping, and diarrhea. Fruit juices are not recommended, as they usually contain a 10 to 15 percent carbohydrate solution.

Luckily for us, sports drink companies read all of this research, too, and formulate sports drinks that have the correct types and concentrations of carbohydrates. So, you can just sit back and enjoy your favorite sports drink without having to worry about the details. For long-duration exercise, an endurance formula may be the way to go. Companies like Gatorade have made endurance formulas that include more electrolytes to help compensate for all of the electrolyte loss that occurs with several hours of training.

Protein: As I discussed in chapter 2, protein is not a major source of energy; only about 10 percent of your energy comes from protein during exercise. Therefore, protein is not a primary consideration during training sessions. Most research does not seem to support any increased benefit from consuming protein during exercise. The one exception to this may be the benefit of obtaining branched-chain amino acids (BCAAs). There is some research to show that BCAAs are metabolized readily during exercise for energy and may help with endurance performance. I will discuss this in more detail in chapter 12. However, at this point, you should focus on carbohydrates and not on protein. If there is a little protein in the carbohydrate-rich food you eat during training, it should not have any negative effects on your training session.

Fat: The recommendations for fat intake may seem a little redundant, but, like the pre-training recommendations, you want to either avoid fats altogether or eat a minimal amount during exercise. Fats will slow down digestion and absorption of other nutrients, and can cause GI problems during training. Small amounts of fat are usually tolerated fairly well for most people during cycling at a low to moderate intensity, but I wouldn't recommend eating fat during high-intensity workouts, or at any time while swimming or running.

Vitamins and Minerals: Consuming electrolytes during training is important if you sweat a lot and during long workouts (ninety minutes or longer). For really long training sessions (those lasting four or more hours), triathletes may need to take some salt tablets or electrolyte tablets. Sodium is the primary electrolyte of concern, and loss of sodium can lead to cramping. The amount of sodium you lose is related to your sweat rate. A triathlete will lose about 1,000 milligrams of sodium per liter of sweat. Therefore, if you calculate your sweat rate, you can estimate your sodium loss as well. Once you have estimated your sodium losses, you can look at the label on your salt tablets and take the proper amount to try to match those losses for your long training session. Remember—if you train for less than four hours, drinking 2

ESTIMATING SODIUM LOSS FROM SWEAT RATES:
An Example

This example is for a five-hour cycling ride:

1. The calculated sweat rate is 24 ounces per hour (3 cups per hour).
2. There are 4.2 cups per liter, so 3 cups of sweat is equal to 0.7 liters.
3. If you lose 1,000 milligrams of sodium per liter of sweat, then 0.7 liters of sweat is equal to 700 milligrams of sodium.
4. Therefore, based on the sweat rate of this triathlete, she loses about 700 milligrams of sodium per hour. The athlete can replenish these losses with sports drinks, salty food, and salt tablets (if needed). Each brand of salt tablet contains a different amount of sodium, so be sure to check the sodium content on the label of each capsule, and do not consume more sodium than your estimated losses.

---

to 4 cups of a sports drink each hour should be sufficient to provide you with the electrolytes that you need.

Post-Training Nutrition

The time immediately following a training session should be thought of as the recovery period. Since triathletes usually exercise daily—and sometimes multiple times within a day—quick and full recovery is crucial. The most important nutrient considerations for recovery are (you guessed it) carbohydrates and fluids, as well as protein.

Carbohydrates: One goal for recovery is to replenish the glycogen stores in your liver and muscles. If glycogen is not replenished after a training session, you will not be adequately fueled when you start your next workout, and your physical performance will most certainly suffer. It is important to replenish glycogen as quickly as possible after exercise. To maximize your body's ability to fully replenish glycogen stores, you need to eat carbohydrates within fifteen to thirty minutes after exercise. This means that high-glycemic-index foods are also recommended right after exercise (foods high in simple sugars). Therefore, during and right after exercise are probably the only two instances where an athlete should try to eat high-glycemic-index foods.

> **Make Note:** To maximize recovery, you should consume carbo-hydrates within fifteen to thirty minutes after exercise. The recommended amount is 1.2 grams of carbohydrates per kilogram of body weight.

The amount of carbohydrate that is needed depends on the length of the workouts. For training sessions that are less than sixty minutes, you only need about 35 to 60 grams of carbohydrates (140 to 240 calories). For sessions lasting longer than ninety minutes (that's actually exercise time, not the time it took to chat with your friends before, during, and after your workout!), you need 1.2 grams of carbohydrates for every kilogram of body weight. This should be consumed immediately after training (within fifteen to thirty minutes), and then again each hour for the next one to four hours (depending on the length of your training session). It can sometimes be challenging to consume this amount of carbs, because you often don't feel like eating right after a hard workout. You should aim for at least 200 calories in that fifteen- to thirty-minute critical window, and then have another meal to get the remaining carbohydrates within two hours after your training session. Liquid calories (recovery drinks, chocolate milk) are often a good choice, because chances are, you'll be more likely to want to drink some-thing right after exercise than to eat a full meal.

Here's how to calculate your calories:

1. Body weight = _____ kilograms

2. Your weight x 1.2 grams per kilogram = _____ grams

3. So, if there are 4 calories per gram of carbohydrates, then _____ grams x 4 calories per gram = _____ calories.

CALCULATING POST-EXERCISE
CARBOHYDRATE INTAKE:
An Example

1. The triathlete weighs 70 kilograms (154 pounds).
2. 70 kilograms x 1.2 grams of carbohydrates per kilogram of body weight = 84 grams of carbohydrates.
3. If there are 4 calories per gram of carbohydrates, then 84 grams of carbohydrates x 4 calories per gram = 336 calories of carbohydrates.

Fluids: It is just as important to replenish fluid losses after exercise as it is during exercise, so you won't be dehydrated for the rest of the day or when you start your next training session. Rehydration should begin immediately after exercise. The best rule of thumb for rehydration is to consume 2 to 3 cups of fluid for each pound lost.

That means you need to weigh yourself before and after you work out (but not in your sweaty clothes). For example, if you lost 2 pounds during your bike ride, then you need to drink 4 to 6 cups of fluid. You should not drink all of these fluids at once. If you have several cups to drink, then spread them out over a three- to five-hour period after exercise.

If you don't have a scale, then you can simply continue drinking fluids until your urine is a pale yellow color. When you are adequately hydrated, you should urinate about one time every one to two hours.

Protein: Protein intake after exercise is important for recovery. It is necessary in order to repair muscle damage and to synthesize new proteins. Just like carbohydrates, there is a critical window in which protein synthesis is maximized. You should consume protein within thirty minutes of your training session. This makes it easy because you can just make sure you get protein and carbohydrates in that first post-exercise meal. You need complete proteins (proteins that contain all essential amino acids), so any animal product (as well as soy) or combination of plant proteins will work. The proper amount of protein is 6 to 20 grams of essential amino acids (which corresponds to 24 to 80 calories). This is a fairly small amount, so whether you've done a forty-five-minute run or a two-hour brick workout (bike ride immediately followed by a transition run), this amount of protein will be adequate to stimulate protein synthesis and repair damaged muscles. If you have just finished exercising for several hours, you need to consume 6 to 20 grams of protein right after exercise, and then just follow your daily protein recommendations for the remainder of the day.

If you've just completed a strength-training or weight-lifting session, then protein intake is critical for protein synthesis and new muscle growth. The type of protein is also more important than the amount. You want to make sure you consume complete proteins (those that contain all nine essential amino acids). Once again, this means getting any animal product or soy (the only plant protein that is complete) or a combination of plant proteins. You should aim for 6 to 20 grams of essential amino acids within thirty minutes of your weight-training session. This is the perfect amount to stimulate protein synthesis and to enhance recovery.

Fat: Replenishing fat after exercise is not important. Even very lean triathletes have relatively large fat reserves. Therefore, unlike carbohydrates and protein, you do not need to replenish the fat you used for energy during exercise. In fact, it is best to minimize the amount of fat you eat right after exercise because it will slow down the digestion and absorption of carbohydrates and protein that your body needs right away. So, keep your first post-exercise meal/drink low in fat (or fat-free). After that, you can simply follow the daily recommendations for fat intake throughout the remainder of the day.

Vitamins and Minerals: If you have been consuming electrolytes during your training session, then you shouldn't have to worry too much about replenishing them after exercise. If you crave salt, you likely don't have enough sodium, so it won't hurt to have electrolytes in your post-exercise meal/drink. You also will have used other vitamins and minerals during exercise (such as B vitamins and antioxidants), but if you follow your daily recommendations for vitamins and minerals, then you shouldn't need to take any extra. If you take one multivitamin/mineral pill each day, you may want to take this pill after a training session. That way, you can use the nutrients in the pill to replenish any that you used during exercise.

Special Considerations

It can be difficult to get food or fluids in during swim workouts, especially if you do open-water swims. Now, on the bright side, most swim workouts don't last more than ninety minutes, regardless of what distance triathlon you train for. That means if you have some fluids available to you (other than pool or lake water), you should be able to meet your nutritional needs. If you swim for longer than one hour, have a sports drink available along with the water. If you do open-water swimming, you may just have to wait until you get out of the water to drink and eat. Now, I have seen some triathletes eat gels during open-water swims, but it looks difficult, and there is nothing to wash it down with. Therefore, I suggest drinking fluids right before and right after the swim.

As I mentioned at the beginning of this chapter, there is a great deal of information to absorb here. The next several chapters will be centered on race-day nutrition for different distances of triathlon races. You may see some recommendations in these chapters that are similar to what you have read about in this one. It is vital to get your nutrition plan down pat during training so you'll know what works best for you on race day.

CHAPTER 8

Sprint and Olympic Triathlons

The Sprint distance triathlon is unique. While it is called a "Sprint," it is also an endurance event, since anything longer than thirty minutes is typically labeled endurance. Sprint triathlon distances vary from race to race, but in general, you're looking at about a 400-meter swim, a 25-kilometer bike (~15 miles), and a 5-kilometer run (3.1 miles). For most triathletes, this type of race will take anywhere from one to two hours to complete. If this is your first triathlon (and it's a good idea to start with a Sprint), then time is not really the issue—crossing the finish line is. In those cases, you will just need to make sure you have prepared your race nutrition for however long it may take.

The Olympic distance triathlon is longer than a Sprint, but it is not the ultra-endurance race that a half or full Ironman is. Some consider it twice as long as a Sprint race, but each discipline may be more or less than twice the Sprint distance race. The distances for this triathlon can also vary from race to race, but the general distances are a 1,500-meter swim (~0.9 miles), a 40-kilometer bike (~25 miles), and a 10-kilometer run (6.2 miles). Most people starting out in the sport of triathlon will start with a Sprint race, but some decide to start with the Olympic distance. Elite athletes can finish an Olympic distance triathlon in about two to two and a half hours, while recreational triathletes may take three to four hours to complete this distance. If this is your first race (or your first race at this distance), your goal may be simply to cross the finish line regardless of the time it takes.

This chapter is designed to provide race-specific nutrition for the Sprint and Olympic distance races. I have combined two different race distances into one chapter because some people will finish a Sprint race in about the same amount of time that it takes others to finish an Olympic distance race. We will start with the twenty-four hours leading up to your event, and then give the exact nutritional information you need right before, during, and after your Sprint or Olympic distance race.

Sprint and Olympic distance races are generally done at higher intensities than other longer races. The higher the intensity of exercise, the more carbohydrates you use for energy. Therefore, carbs are very important both before and during a Sprint and Olympic distance triathlon because they are what your body uses as its primary source of energy.

I do say "high-intensity" with some caution, though. While working with a friend of mine on his race nutrition for shorter-distance races, I asked him why he wasn't drinking or eating much on the bike. His response? "I can't eat or drink because then I can't breathe." If you are going so hard that you physically lose your breath, or can't afford to spare one second to swallow because you are so out of breath, you probably are going just a little too hard. When I didn't respond immediately to my friend and let his words sort of hang in the air between us, he finally started laughing as he realized how crazy that sounded. The moral of the story? Even though these races are done at a higher intensity, keep in mind that you still need to be able to breathe and eat and drink.

Twenty-Four Hours Before the Race

Most races begin early in the morning, so here I'm basically talking about what you're going to eat the day before your event. I know what you're thinking: "Does it really matter what I eat the day before my race?" The answer is yes. What you eat the day before actually does have an impact on your race-day performance. People always think that their nutrition the day before a race doesn't really matter unless they're doing an ultra-endurance event, but they are wrong. While your nutrition the day before an event may not impact whether or not you finish a race of this distance, it can definitely affect your overall performance in the race.

The day before your race, you want to stick with foods that you are used to eating; you should never try something that you haven't had before. This can be difficult if you have traveled for your race and are eating out at restaurants. If that is the case, at least order things that seem relatively "safe," such as salads and sandwiches.

Now let's talk about what you need, and then what you want to avoid or minimize.

Focus on Carbohydrates: Your focus should still be on carbohydrates, as that is your primary energy source. While you will not likely deplete your glycogen/carbohydrate stores during this distance race (although you could during an Olympic distance event), you want to make sure your glycogen stores are "topped off" before the event. Therefore, you want to get about 55 to 60 percent of your calories from carbohydrates, about 15 to 20 percent from protein, and about 20 to 30 percent from fat. These recommendations are similar to what you should be eating on a regular basis (see chapter 1 for a refresher on recommendations), although the fat recommendation is a little lower.

I have found that most athletes feel better when they wake up on race morning if they have had a slightly lower fat intake the previous day, especially from the evening meal. Therefore, if you eat a big pasta dinner the night before your event, make sure it is not loaded with fat (meaning, avoid the cream sauces, and don't eat too much buttery garlic bread). If you're not sure what to eat, follow the sample meal plans that I have included in the appendix for day-to-day nutrition. You may need to make a few modifications (i.e., lower the fat and fiber), but the plans should help you with planning your pre-race nutrition, especially if you are someone who does not want to count grams of carbohydrates, fat, and protein to see if you fall within the correct percentages.

Don't Forget about Fiber: In addition to lowering your fat intake slightly, there are a couple of other nutrients or foods you want to eat less of. One of those is fiber. Normally, I am a huge proponent of fiber. It has numerous health benefits, and most people don't get enough of it in their diets, so I always push athletes to consume more fiber. However, fiber does delay digestion and absorption of other nutrients, pulls a great deal of water into the intestines, and can cause some acute GI distress (such as gas, cramping, and bloating). It also takes longer to "clear the system" than other types of carbohydrates. This means that eating a lot of fiber the day before an event can actually have detrimental effects on race day. Therefore, you should lower your fiber intake in the twenty-four hours before your race.

There is no recommended amount of fiber that I can suggest because it all depends on your usual intake. For example, if you consume 20 grams of fiber per day, but your fellow triathlete friend consumes about 10 grams of fiber per day, recommending 15 grams of fiber in the twenty-four hours before a race is good advice for you, but not for your friend. Fiber is important, and you should aim to intake the recommended amounts (30 to 38 grams per day for men, and 21 to 25 grams per day for women). Cut back the fiber about 25 to 35 percent the day before your race, and you should be just fine.

If you don't really want to get into counting grams of fiber in your diet, then here are some simple rules to follow:

1. Eat less whole grains (choose white bread, bagels, tortillas, and rice, instead of brown).

2. Cut back on fiber-rich vegetables (avocado, broccoli, Brussels sprouts, cabbage, carrots, chickpeas, and mushrooms).

3. Limit bran and beans (such as navy, kidney, pinto, black, lima, and white).

4. Cut back on fiber-rich fruits (apples, bananas, and berries such as blueberries, blackberries, and raspberries).

I know these things all sound counterintuitive to everything you've heard about eating healthy, but remember—you're trying to cut back on the fiber for just one day.

Limit the Sodium and Sugar: Another thing you may want to limit the day before your event is foods that are really high in sodium or sugar. This is especially true for the evening before one of these shorter-distance races. Although sodium is very important for endurance athletes, you typically get plenty of sodium in your diet already, and you will not lose huge amounts during these race distances. Sodium causes water retention, so triathletes who eat sodium-rich foods the evening before a race tend to wake up feeling bloated, heavier, and extremely thirsty. High-sugar foods tend to have the same effect. Therefore, in order to avoid waking up feeling like you have a hangover, try not to overdo it with the salt and sugar the evening before your race. This can be difficult if you eat out in a restaurant, as eateries tend to serve food with large amounts of sodium. However, you can always ask the restaurant to hold back on the salt, or choose items that you know will not be quite as salty, such as eating dinner rolls instead of garlic bread, or a chicken breast, vegetables, and rice or sweet potato instead of spaghetti with a salty sauce like marinara.

Remember the Fluids: The fluid recommendations for the day before a race do not change from your everyday recommendations (see chapter 6 for a review). To ensure that you are properly hydrated, drink plenty of water throughout the day. If you don't want to count cups of water, then you can use urination as a guide. When you are properly hydrated, your urine should be pale yellow, and you should urinate once every one to two hours. If you follow this guideline (or your actual fluid recommendations), you can be reassured that you will be hydrated for your race. As for micronutrient intake, there are no vitamins or minerals that you need extra amounts of; just consume your normal daily amounts (take your multivitamin/mineral if that is what you do every day), and you will be just fine.

Pre-Race Nutrition

Pre-race nutrition covers the four hours before the start of your race. Most races start pretty early in the morning, so it's really important to make sure that you get up early enough not only to eat your pre-race meal, but also to allow enough time for digestion and absorption of that meal to occur. For this meal, focus on a lot of carbohydrates, a small amount of protein, and little to no fat. Here are the specifics:

Carbohydrates: Recommended intake is 1.0 to 3.5 grams per kilogram of body weight in the one to four hours before the race. This is a pretty broad recommendation mainly because the amount of time that you eat this meal before a race affects how much you should eat. I recommend that you eat your pre-race meal two to three hours before the gun goes off. This will give you enough time to digest and absorb your meal so that you will not have to worry about GI distress during your race. If you eat four hours before

> **Make Note:** Eat your pre-race meal two to three hours before the gun goes off so you have time to digest and absorb all the nutrients.

the event, you may get hungry by the time your race starts, and you do not want to start a race feeling hungry (that's an indication that you have done something wrong).

You also don't want to eat too much within two hours of your race because it is unlikely that the food will be completely digested and absorbed. This sets you up for some GI distress during your race. The intensity of the race also needs to be factored in. Since the Sprint and Olympic distance triathlons are usually higher in intensity than some of the longer-distance triathlons, aiming for the low end of the carbohydrate recommendation is warranted. Therefore, if you eat two to three hours before the race, you should consume about 1.5 to 2.0 grams of carbohydrate per kilogram of body weight.

Here is how to do your own calculation:

1. Lower end of the range: Your weight (in kilograms): _____ x 1.5 grams = _____ grams of carbohydrate.

2. Upper end of the range: Your weight (in kilograms): _____ x 2.0 grams = _____ grams of carbohydrate.

3. There are 4 calories per gram of carbohydrate, so this meal equates to _____ to _____ calories of carbohydrate (_____ to _____ grams x 4 calories per gram for carbohydrate).

CALCULATING YOUR PRE-RACE CARBOHYDRATE INTAKE: An Example

1. Triathlete who weighs 80 kilograms (176 pounds).
2. Lower end of the range: 80 kilograms x 1.5 grams of carbohydrate = 120 grams of carbohydrate.
3. Upper end of the range: 80 kilograms x 2.0 grams of carbohydrate = 160 grams of carbohydrate.
4. There are 4 calories per gram of carbohydrate, so this meal will contain 480 to 800 calories of carbohydrate (120 grams x 4 calories per gram = 480 calories and 160 grams x 4 calories per gram = 640 calories).

The type of carbohydrate is also important. You want to minimize fiber in order to reduce potential GI distress, and you also want to minimize high amounts of sugar. Instead, consume complex carbohydrates that are easily digested and have a low glycemic index (low to moderate levels of sugar). I discussed in chapter 7 why you do not want high-sugar foods right before exercising, and the same rule applies to before competition. High-sugar foods cause a rapid rise in blood glucose levels. This leads to a large insulin response, which lowers blood glucose levels. Low blood glucose levels during exercise decrease performance and can cause feelings of hypoglycemia. In the appendix I provide some pre-race meals that contain the proper amounts and types of carbohydrates.

Protein: There is very little research on whether or not protein consumed before competition can help with performance. Most of the research that points toward some benefits has been done in ultra-endurance events. For a Sprint or Olympic distance triathlon, you will not use much protein for energy, so protein intake before competition is not nearly as important as carbohydrate intake. There are some benefits to getting protein in your pre-race meal, though, one of which is the satiating effect of protein (it helps you feel full right after a meal). Protein can take longer to digest and absorb than carbohydrates, so you don't want to eat too much in your pre-race meal. Stick to about 6 to 20 grams of protein in the meal (24 to 80 calories) that you're eating about two to three hours before your race. You should always practice your pre-race meal during a training day, so if you can tolerate more protein, feel free; just make sure you don't eat more protein at the expense of carbohydrates.

Fat: There is very little place for fat when you start discussing race nutrition. Fat is the nutrient that takes the longest to digest and absorb, and also tends to cause the most GI distress. Every triathlete also has plenty of fat stores, so you don't need to worry about depleting yourself of this energy reserve. Even the leanest athlete stores thousands of calories of fat that can be used for energy at any time. Therefore, for the pre-race meal, you should either completely avoid fat or consume it in small amounts. Some triathletes are able to tolerate fat quite well, while others cannot handle any fat. If your pre-race meal has some fat (less than 10 grams) and you've practiced with that before, then you should be all set. It is actually hard to find a pre-race meal that does not contain any fat, so you will likely eat at least a few grams.

Make Note: Your pre-race meal should either be fat-free or contain small amounts of fat (less than 10 grams for the whole meal). This will help prevent GI distress during the race.

Fluids: When you get up on race morning, the first thing you should think about is rehydrating from your eight-hour fast during sleeping. (I know; I'm probably being overly optimistic that you got eight hours of sleep—espe cially if you're nervous.) You should drink 1 to 2 cups of fluid when you first wake up (this should be about four hours before your race). Two hours before the start of your race, you should drink an additional cup of fluid. Finally, twenty to thirty minutes before the start of the race, drink one more cup of fluid. Some people get a side ache when they drink right before high-intensity exercise. If that's you, make sure you allow thirty minutes before the start of the race when you drink that last cup of fluids. Some triathletes prefer to sip water or other fluids all during the pre-race hours instead of drinking entire cups of fluid at a given time. This is fine to do as long as you consume the same amount of fluids as what is recommended here.

Make Note: Pre-race fluid intake: Drink 1 to 2 cups when you first wake up, 1 cup two hours before the race, and 1 cup twenty to thirty minutes before the race.

The type of fluid depends a great deal on personal preference. Water is the best choice, and sports drinks can be a good alternative. However, remember that sports drinks are pretty much all sugar, so don't drink too much of those in that last hour before your race because you don't want to disrupt your blood glucose levels too much. You can get some of your fluids from coffee or tea, but keep in mind that they usually have caffeine. Since caffeine is a diuretic, you will not retain all of that fluid you consume. Moderate amounts of caffeine do not really have any ergogenic effects on performance, but if you are used to getting your caffeine fix each morning, then do not deprive yourself of caffeine on race day. That will do more harm than good. You will likely feel lethargic, tired, and irritable, and neither you nor your competitors want that.

Some drinks to avoid, however, are carbonated beverages. These typically cause some GI distress and are not tolerated well with exercise. Some triathletes also try to avoid milk before a race, as it can cause GI distress for some people and also leaves a filmy/mucus-like taste in your mouth. Finally, juices are generally not recommended unless they are consumed in the two- to four-hour period before your race. Their sugar concentration is usually twice as high as that of sports drinks, so they can really affect your blood glucose concentrations.

During-Race Nutrition

Your nutrition during a race really depends on how long it takes you to do your Sprint or Olympic distance triathlon. Many triathletes can finish a Sprint race in one to one and a half hours. If this is you, then your nutrition plan will be fairly simple. However, if it takes you longer than that, or if you do the Olympic distance race, then we need to make sure you have thoroughly planned out your race nutrition.

Athletes Racing for Ninety Minutes or Less

I will start with those triathletes who will finish a Sprint in one to one and a half hours. The nutritional concerns for these athletes are carbohydrates and fluids. You do not need any protein or fat (and really should avoid it in order to prevent GI complications). You also should not have to worry about replacing electrolytes, since you're racing for such a short period of time.

Carbohydrates: For exercise lasting sixty minutes or less, no carbohydrates are necessary. The sixty- to ninety-minute window is a bit of a gray area, though, so if it only takes you an hour, then you really do not need any additional carbohydrates. If you will finish your race closer to the ninety-minute mark, I recommend consuming some carbohydrates. The carbohydrate recommendation is 60 to 70 grams per hour. If you will race for ninety minutes, then I recommend consuming about 30 grams of carbohydrate around minute thirty of the race, and then another 15 to 30 grams of carbohydrate at about the one-hour mark. For Sprint triathlons I recommend all calories come from fluids or gels. The nature of the race dictates a very high intensity, and liquid and gel calories are just easier for the body to handle.

That first 30 grams of carbohydrate can easily be consumed with one gel (they usually have about 20 to 25 grams of carbohydrate) and a little bit of a sports drink (each cup usually has 15 grams of carbohydrate). If this is consumed at minute thirty, you should be on your bike. It is usually easiest to eat during the bike portion of the race, so consume that gel and a little bit of your favorite sports drink (¼ to ½ cup) and you will be all set. If you prefer specialty sports drinks that are more concentrated, then it is possible to get all 30 grams of carbohydrate from that. Just make sure you know how much carbohydrate is in your specialty drink so you will know how much to consume. The second (and optional) point of caloric intake is at minute sixty. This will likely be at the start of your run or partway into your run. If you are running fast, then it may be hard to consume anything other than liquid calories. If you consume 1 cup of a popular sports drink, you will get the amount of carbohydrate that you need.

Fluids: Fluids are the other nutritional concern. You want to aim to intake about 1 cup of fluid every twenty minutes, but you need to keep in mind that this is a short, intense race, and you will likely not exercise long enough to really suffer from dehydration. Therefore, some triathletes only take in about 2 cups total for this distance race. Since you do not need much (or any) carbohydrate, then water is the best choice.

If you plan to get some carbohydrates from fluids, then you will want to drink sports drinks and water. Again, since Sprint races are usually high-intensity, you want to consume fluids early on, during the bike portion, so that you don't end up with a side ache during your run. It is best to limit or avoid fluids in that last fifteen minutes on the bike before you start your run. By doing this, you won't feel like you have a lot of liquid sloshing around in your stomach when you start running. Then, during the run, you can consume a small amount of fluid (½ cup) to get you to the finish line.

Athletes Racing for Ninety Minutes or Longer

Now I will focus on those triathletes who will be racing for ninety minutes to four-plus hours. The nutrition is very similar for either the Sprint or Olympic distance races, as long as they fall within that ninety-minute to four-plus-hour window. Your primary nutritional concerns are carbohydrates and fluids. Protein is not necessary, although small amounts will likely not have a negative effect on your performance. Fat is not necessary and can cause GI distress, so try to avoid it during your race.

Carbohydrates: You will need carbohydrates during your race. The recommended amount is 60 to 70 grams per hour, and you should begin this soon after the onset of the race. It is difficult to eat anything during the swim portion of the race, so your eating will likely begin on the bike. It usually works out pretty well for triathletes to eat about 30 grams of carbohydrates every thirty minutes. Again, this can be achieved with a gel and/or a sports drink or a specialty drink. Look at the nutrition-facts panel of your food and fluids before your race, and set up your nutrition plan so you know exactly what to consume in order to get that 30 grams every thirty minutes. If you get on your bike fifteen minutes into the race, then you will have a little time to settle in before you need to eat.

For the Olympic distances, you will likely get out of the water somewhere near the thirty-minute mark (or later). Therefore, you should try to take in that initial 30 grams of carbohydrates very soon after you start biking. Sometimes triathletes are out of breath from transition, so wait about 1 mile so that you will be settled into your bike pace before eating. If you plan on eating some solid foods as well as liquids, I recommend eating the solid foods early on during the bike portion, and then switching over to gels and liquids for the end of the bike and the run portions of the race. Regardless of the source, continue to eat carbohydrates every thirty minutes until the finish.

Fluids: Fluid recommendations are the same as those above: about 1 cup every twenty minutes. Again, you should limit or avoid fluids in the last fifteen minutes on the bike so you don't feel like you have a stomach full of liquids when you start running. If it is hot and/or humid and you sweat a lot, you can have significant electrolyte losses. Therefore, I recommend that you consume both water and sports drinks (which contain electrolytes) to replace some of those losses. Incidentally, most other sports-nutrition products do have electrolytes in them, so if you eat a gel, you will get some electrolytes. I will discuss salt tablets in upcoming chapters, but if you race for four-plus hours, then you may need one or two electrolyte tablets (shoot for about 250 to 450 milligrams total from tablets). The appendix provides some examples of food and fluid intake for both Sprint and Olympic distance races.

Post-Race Nutrition

First off, congratulate yourself on finishing your race. Whether this is your first triathlon or you've done one hundred Sprint or Olympic distance races, it's always an accomplishment to cross the finish line. Never forget that. So many athletes get really caught up in the competitiveness of the race (which, don't get me wrong, is great—I'm quite competitive myself) that they forget to enjoy it and be happy when they finish. Now that you've patted yourself on the back, let's get down to the nuts and bolts of your post-race nutrition.

Probably one of the last things you want to do right after your race is to think about nutrition, but it is really important for recovery. And recovery is crucial, because you most likely will do another race in the future, which means you probably will get right back to training.

Your goals for recovery are to:

1. Replenish glycogen.

2. Provide protein for muscle function/repair/rebuilding.

3. Rehydrate.

If you remember nothing else about recovery nutrition, remember the fifteen- to thirty-minute critical window. The three recovery processes I just mentioned are all working at their peak right after your race. Therefore, you need to provide the correct nutrients during that fifteen- to thirty-minute window of time. Let's start with carbohydrates.

Make Note: Recovery nutrition begins immediately after racing. Begin post-race nutrition within that fifteen- to thirty-minute critical window in order to maximum recovery.

Carbohydrates: The recommended amount of carbohydrates to consume post-race is 1.2 grams per kilogram of body weight. Since most triathletes do not feel like eating right after a race (especially if it was a high-intensity race), liquid calories are an excellent choice. You also want to consume high-glycemic-index carbohydrates (higher amounts of sugar). These foods are digested and absorbed more quickly, and speed is what you need at this point. Some examples and post-race meals are shown in the appendix (see pages 177–81).

Here is how to do your own post-race nutrition recommendation calculation (I've provided an example calculation for a triathlete, and space for you to do your own):

1. Your weight (in kilograms): _____ x 1.2 grams = _____ grams of carbohydrate.

2. Since there are 4 calories for each gram of carbohydrate, this equates to _____ calories of carbohydrate (_____ grams x 4 calories per gram for carbohydrate).

CALCULATING POST-RACE CARBOHYDRATE INTAKE: An Example

1. This triathlete weighs 80 kilograms (176 pounds): 80 kilograms x 1.2 grams of carbohydrate = 96 grams of carbohydrates.
2. There are 4 calories per gram of carbohydrate, so this meal will contain 384 calories of carbohydrate (96 grams x 4 calories per gram = 384 calories).

Even if you consume liquid calories, this amount of carbohydrate can be difficult for some triathletes to handle right after a race. If you are one of those people, try and get some calories in, and then consume another meal rich in carbohydrates one to two hours later.

Protein: Protein is important right after exercise for repair and rebuilding of tissue. Protein synthesis can be increased anywhere from 10 to 90 percent after endurance exercise. You do not need much, though; 6 to 20 grams (24 to 80 calories) of protein is the recommended amount. More than that will not be harmful, but it will not lead to any additional protein synthesis or quicker recovery. The type of protein is quite important. You want to be sure you get all of your essential amino acids. These complete proteins (which contain all nine essential amino acids) can be found in any animal product, as well as soy. All other plant proteins will be missing at least one essential amino acid.

Fluids: Fluids are the other major nutritional concern post-race. Even if you follow the fluid recommendations for your race, you will end your race slightly dehydrated. Therefore, start drinking fluids right after you've completed your race. During training, you can weigh yourself before and after exercise sessions and rehydrate accordingly (2 to 3 cups of fluid for every pound lost). However, I doubt you will have a scale available after your Sprint or Olympic distance race, so you will just have to estimate it.

Start drinking fluids—and keep drinking periodically—throughout the first two hours of recovery, until you are rehydrated (physical signs will be that your urine is pale yellow and you urinate every one to two hours). Then you can simply follow your regular fluid recommendations for the remainder of the day.

Fat: As I mentioned above, you won't deplete your fat stores during this race (sorry to disappoint). Therefore, replenishing fat is not critical. However, most foods do have some fat in them. It's just fine to consume small amounts of fat right after your race; keep in mind, though, that fat does slow down digestion and absorption of other nutrients. Because of this, you do not want a lot of fat in your post-race meal, since it is vitally important to get those carbs and protein digested and absorbed quickly. Also, try to stick to MUFAs and PUFAs, which are healthy fats, and limit SFAs and trans fats, the unhealthy fats (see pages 26–28).

Vitamins and Minerals: Similarly, you do not need to worry about specific micronutrient replacement. If you eat a healthy diet for the remainder of the day, then you will get the nutrients that you need. If you crave salt, then listen to your body. You may have lost more sodium through sweat than you were able to replace, and your body may need a little more.

There are a number of recovery drinks available on the market. Personally, I'm a huge proponent of chocolate milk. Research studies have shown that chocolate milk equals (or even exceeds) some specially designed recovery drinks, and it's also easier on the budget. Chocolate milk seems to provide just the right amount of carbs and protein, it's in liquid form, and it doesn't have too much fat (as long as you stick to the low-fat variety; otherwise, it can have quite a bit of fat). Some other recovery options can be found in the appendix.

The post-race meal that you consume fifteen to thirty minutes after your race is the most important for you, but it is also crucial to keep that recovery process going for the rest of the day. In order to do that, you need to eat a healthy diet and provide your body with the nutrients it needs. Consume a carbohydrate-rich meal one to two hours after your race (especially if you did not get 1.2 grams of carbohydrates per kilogram of body weight in that first post-race meal). Added to that meal should be some complete proteins and fluids. After that, simply focus on a healthy diet for the rest of the day.

CHAPTER 9

Half Ironman Triathlon

W hen you start getting into distances like the half Ironman, proper nutrition is not only important, it is essential for your performance. My friend Sam, who slowed considerably during his half Ironman race, can attest to the fact that you need more (way more) than 2 to 3 cups of water and a couple hundred calories for your race. You may be able to finish the race on that amount (he did finish), but I don't think he appreciated having hundreds of people run past him while he suffered through the run.

If you are like most other triathletes, you spend a good deal of time planning out your training for this event (or your coach has spent a good deal of time on your training program). Similarly, you have probably planned out every detail of your half Ironman race, right down to the color towel you use in transition. However, if I were to ask you what your specific nutrition plan was for the day before the event, as well as during and after the event, what would you say? If you're like most triathletes I know, your answer would be something very vague about your plan for the twenty-four hours leading up to the race. You also probably have a general plan of taking in some food (probably gels, bloks, or bars) and some fluids (water, and whatever else is available on the course). However, if you haven't mapped out your nutrition down to detailed amounts, then you're not preparing properly. Spend the time planning out your nutrition; you will thank yourself for it later.

Twenty-Four Hours Before the Race

If what you eat is important before a Sprint or Olympic distance race, then it's obviously important for a half Ironman. The recommendations are very similar to those of other race distances, so you may notice some overlap between chapter 8 and this chapter. Your main focus should be on carbohydrate intake, followed closely by fluids. One of the biggest differences between a race of this distance and a Sprint or Olympic distance race is that you will become glycogen-depleted during a half Ironman if you do not take in the proper amount of carbohydrates. Therefore, the more carbs you can store in your body before the race, the better.

In chapter 1 on carbohydrates, I discussed two different methods for glycogen or carbohydrate loading. The half Ironman distance is a perfect distance for loading if you decide to go that route. Sprint and Olympic distance triathlons are usually too short (meaning you won't get much additional benefit from glycogen loading because you're not depleting your carbohydrate stores during those races). Conversely, the full Ironman is too long. You would get some benefit from loading, but even with carbohydrate loading, there will still be several hours when you race without glycogen stores in reserve. Therefore, if you are interested in carbohydrate loading, I suggest you do it for this distance race. If that is the route you're going to take, then follow the glycogen-loading protocols from chapter 1 (see pages 12–15) instead of the following nutrition information.

> **Make Note:** The half Ironman is the perfect distance race for carbohydrate or glycogen loading.

Remember that carbohydrates are our primary energy source, and you want to at least top off glycogen levels (even if you aren't planning on following a loading protocol). Therefore, about 60 to 65 percent of your calories should come from carbohydrates. This is slightly higher than the recommended percentage for Sprint and Olympic distance races, because having more carbohydrates available is more important for this race. Fifteen to 20 percent of your calories should be coming from protein, and the remaining calories should be coming from fat (20 to 25 percent). You should also follow the normal daily fluid recommendations from chapter 6. If you're worried that you may not get enough water, then add a cup or two to that total for the day before your race. You can also drink a cup of water before bed, since it will be several hours before you drink again; however, this may backfire by causing you to wake up in the middle of the night for a bathroom break.

The types of carbohydrates, proteins, and fats that you should eat are similar to that before a sprint or Olympic distance race.

Here's a refreshers of the do's and don'ts:

Summary of Nutrition Tips for 24-Hours Pre-Race

1. Do focus on complex carbohydrates, complete proteins (those that contain all of your essential amino acids, such as meats, soy, or combinations of plant proteins), and healthy fats.

2. Do eat a carbohydrate- and protein-rich dinner the evening before the race.

3. Do aim for a low-fat dinner the evening before the race, a maximum of 15 percent of total calories from that meal coming from fat —with as many of those fat calories being MUFAs and PUFAs rather than SFAs. If you're unsure what type of fat it is, most fats from plant products are healthier that those from animal products.

4. Don't eat a lot of fiber the day before your race. I recommend for this distance race that you cut back on your daily fiber by about 30 to 50 percent of your usual intake. This means that if you usually eat about 30 grams of fiber, then aim for 15 to 20 grams the day before your race. To help cut back on fiber, choose "white"—this means white bread, white rice, and/or white pasta. Also, cut back on beans and vegetables, especially with your evening meal.

5. Do get an adequate amount of vitamins and minerals the day before your race (you will accomplish this if you eat a healthy diet, and/or if you take a multivitamin/mineral pill).

6. Don't eat too much sodium (salt) the night before your race. This tends to make athletes feel thirsty and bloated on race morning. Instead, try to eat a fairly high-sodium diet in the days leading up to your race, and earlier during the day before your race. Just cut back some on dinner so you don't feel sluggish on race morning.

7.   Don't eat a lot of high-sugar foods such as desserts and candy the night before your race. Trust me, you'll get enough sugary foods during your race; you can lay off them the night before.

In general, if you eat a healthy diet on a daily basis, you really don't need to change your eating habits very much on the day before your race.

Pre-Race Nutrition

To get your pre-race meal digested and absorbed, you need to get up at least three to four hours before your race. You should eat your pre-race meal three hours before your race, so get up early enough to have a little bit of an appetite. If this is your first half Ironman, you will probably be nervous. The last thing you will want to do is eat, but you need to force yourself to get your breakfast down. Just think of it as part of your race plan. You wouldn't skip pumping up your bike tires, so don't skip this meal. Additionally, the first thing you should do when you wake up is drink 8 to 16 ounces of water, because you haven't had any fluids all night.

Carbohydrates: Your pre-race meal should be carbohydrate-rich, with some protein and just a little bit of fat. You should aim for 2 to 3 grams of carbohydrate per kilogram of body weight. This is higher than the amount for a Sprint or Olympic distance race, so practice with this before some of your long rides and/or runs to make sure you can tolerate this amount.

Here is how to calculate your own intake:

1.   Lower end of the range: Your weight (in kilograms): _____
      x 2.0 grams = _____ grams of carbohydrate. Since there are 4
      calories for each gram of carbohydrate, this equates to _____
      calories of carbohydrate (your gram number x 4).

2.   Upper end of the range: Your weight (in kilograms): _____
      x 3.0 grams = _____ grams of carbohydrate. Since there are 4
      calories for each gram of carbohydrate, this equates to _____
      calories of carbohydrate (your gram number x 4). Range of
      carbohydrate calories for the meal is _____ to _____ .

CALCULATING YOUR PRE-RACE CARBOHYDRATE INTAKE: An Example

This triathlete weighs 80 kilograms (176 pounds).

1. Lower end of range: 80 kilograms x 2.0 grams of carbohydrate = 160 grams of carbohydrate. Since there are 4 calories per gram of carbohydrate, this would be 480 calories of carbohydrate (160 grams x 4 calories per gram = 640 calories).
2. Upper end of range: 80 kilograms x 3.0 grams of carbohydrate = 240 grams of carbohydrate. Since there are 4 calories per gram of carbohydrate, this would be 960 calories (240 grams x 4 calories per gram = 960 calories). Therefore, this meal will contain between 480 to 960 calories of carbohydrate.

Remember that you want to keep this meal low in fiber, but you don't want it to be all simple sugars— especially if you eat anything within one hour of your race (we're aiming for low glycemic index here). You can refer to the appendix for some sample pre-race meal ideas.

Protein: Just like with a Sprint or Olympic distance triathlon, you will not use a lot of protein for energy. However, it won't hurt to get a little protein in your pre-race meal. Try to get about 6 to 20 grams of protein; much higher than that, and your pre-race meal starts to get too large. Since you do not want a lot of fat at this meal, stick to lean protein sources.

Fat: You want to keep fat fairly low at this meal. Now, if you eat three hours before your race, that should be plenty of time to digest and absorb all of your food, but if it is a high-fat meal, that may not be the case. If you are someone who has GI problems when racing, keep fat out of this meal altogether, or consume as little as possible. For those of you with tougher stomachs, you can go as high as 15 percent of calories from this meal as fat.

Fluids: Next to carbohydrates, fluids are the most important nutrient on race morning. You should drink 1 to 2 cups of water upon waking (about three to four hours before your race). Drink 1 more cup of fluid two hours before your race, and then another cup about thirty minutes before your race. Alternatively, you can sip fluids throughout your pre-race period; just make sure you get at least 3 to 4 cups in the four-hour pre-race period. I recommend water for most of the fluids (especially the cup you drink thirty minutes before the race). You should not drink anything with high sugar (such as juice or a sports drink) within thirty minutes of the start of your race; this is because you do not want to have a spike in blood glucose followed by a crash just as your race is starting. It's up to you to decide what type of fluids you drink two and four hours before the race. If you want to drink juice to get some of your carbohydrate calories with your pre-race meal, that is fine.

Finally, if you usually drink coffee or tea on a daily basis, do the same thing on race day. While caffeine is a diuretic, if you drink water in addition to your cup of joe, you probably won't be dehydrated at the start of your race (and you won't have a pounding headache from caffeine withdrawal).

During-Race Nutrition

Hopefully you've practiced your nutrition during your long rides and runs. If you have been doing this correctly, then you don't need to change anything for race day. For a race of this distance, you should be thinking about the Big Three: carbohydrates, fluids, and electrolytes (sodium in particular).

> **Make Note:** Although 60 to 70 grams of carbohydrate per hour works for shorter distances, up to 90 grams of carbs per hour is optimal for a race of this distance.

Carbohydrates: The more carbohydrates your body can handle, the better (up to a certain point). From previous chapters, we have learned that 60 to 70 grams per hour is the target. This seems to be the best amount for races up to about two and a half hours in length. However, more and more research shows that for races longer than three hours, up to 90 grams of carbohydrate per hour is optimal. Since you have done this in training, you will know what your body can tolerate. Some athletes can handle up to 90 grams per hour, including a few familiar names (Lance Armstrong and Chrissie Wellington reportedly handle this amount without problems). So, if you are lucky enough to be able to tolerate up to 90 grams per hour, then shoot for that. You should not go above this amount, however; if you do, you will almost certainly experience some GI distress. In addition, your body will not be able to digest and absorb it quickly enough to utilize it anyway.

If you seem to be able to handle only about 40 to 45 grams per hour, you are not alone. Some triathletes simply cannot handle more carbohydrates than that. Now, increasing your amount is trainable, and I have discussed ways to train your body to tolerate more carbohydrates in chapter 7. The only way people can handle up to 90 grams per hour of carbohydrate is if the carbs are a combination of glucose and fructose. Fructose alone will cause GI distress, but when combined with glucose, those complications tend to go away. Nearly all of the sports-nutrition products will contain the best ratio or combination of glucose to fructose in order to maximize absorption and utilization in the body. If you don't want to consume gels or other sports-nutrition products, you probably won't know the exact ratio of glucose to fructose that you consume, but you can still focus on the total amount of carbohydrates to make sure you stick to the recommendations. Most foods that you eat will have both glucose and fructose in them if they are sweet/sugary products. In fact, anything that lists sucrose (table sugar) in the ingredient list will be providing both glucose and fructose.

You should consume carbohydrates periodically throughout each hour rather than eating all 60 to 70 grams at once. Since you probably won't eat anything during the swim, you will need to start taking in carbohydrates soon after starting the bike portion of your race. I recommend waiting until about mile two or three before eating anything. This is simply because some athletes go into the red zone (meaning, a high intensity that cannot be sustained for long periods of time) during their transition, and it takes a mile or two to get into your cycling rhythm. Once you start taking in carbs on the bike, continue to follow the plan you devised before the race to be sure you get them in frequently.

Sometimes it's easy to remember to eat during training rides, but for some reason triathletes tend to forget all about eating and drinking when race day comes. A friend of mine actually sets a timer on her watch to go off every ten minutes to remind her to drink, and a second reminder goes off every thirty minutes to remind her to eat 30 to 35 grams of carbohydrates. If you tend to forget to eat or drink, give that a try.

You do not want to start the run portion of your race with a full stomach. Try to plan out your nutrition so you eat your last amount of carbohydrates at least fifteen minutes before you start running. Then you should start eating about fifteen minutes into your run (assuming you're following a plan that involves 30 to 35 grams of carbohydrates every thirty minutes). Also, don't shortchange yourself toward the end of the race. If you are scheduled to take a gel but only have one or two miles left, don't skip it. It's not worth the dollar you will save on the product if you run out of gas and have to drag yourself to the finish line.

Fluids: Preventing or delaying dehydration for a half or full Ironman race is imperative. Nothing will slow you down more on race day than dehydration. Just ask any triathlete who is on the side of the road during race day, trying to stretch out because of muscle cramps. Now, cramping doesn't occur only because of dehydration, but it is a major culprit. Start drinking fluids as soon as you get on the bike. You have most likely just finished swimming hard for twenty to fifty minutes, so you're a little behind on your fluid intake by the time you start biking. (Drinking lake water by accident does not count as fluid intake.) Just like with carbohydrates, you may want to wait until miles two or three before you start drinking in order to quickly get into your cycling rhythm.

If you performed a sweat trial during a training bike ride and a training run, you should know how much fluid you need each hour (see chapter 6 for a review). Triathletes can absorb about 1 liter (4.2 cups) of fluid easily on the bike, but only about 500 milliliters of fluid during the run. Therefore, if your sweat rate was 6 or 7 cups per hour, you won't be able to match that. Try to get at least 4 cups per hour to delay dehydration, or to at least lessen its severity. Since you can absorb about 4 cups per hour while biking, you should drink about 1 cup every fifteen minutes. Some triathletes can sustain that amount on the run. If you are one of those lucky ones, keep drinking 1 cup every fifteen minutes on the run. If you tend to get side aches or feel your stomach distend because you're not absorbing the fluids, you will have to back off. Try drinking 1 cup of fluid every twenty minutes instead (or a half-cup every ten to fifteen minutes). Hopefully you have done some practice rides and runs at an intensity that is close to your race pace so that you know what your body can handle.

For fluids, the go-to source is water and sports drinks. You will need electrolytes during a race of this distance, which is why sports drinks are recommended (they also provide some carbohydrates). Many of the triathletes I advise consume a mixture of water and sports drinks. If you consume a specialty formula, make sure you know what is in it. It may contain large amounts of carbohydrate, which, if consumed in addition to food, may give you too many carbohydrates and calories. Stay away from juices (unless you dilute them) because they have too high a concentration of carbohydrates.

Electrolytes: You do not need to concern yourself with any other vitamins and minerals other than electrolytes. Furthermore, the only electrolyte you really need to focus on is sodium. You will almost always get chloride with your sodium, and you do not want to get huge amounts of potassium because it can cause heart arrhythmias. You should never take a potassium pill for just this reason. Most sports drinks and sports-nutrition products contain large amounts of sodium and modest amounts of potassium and chloride. While you need to replace all three of these electrolytes, sodium should be your main concern.

If you sweat a lot or if you're racing in a hot, humid environment, you may need some electrolyte tablets/pills in addition to sports-nutrition products. Salt tablets are recommended for triathletes racing longer than four hours (or three hours in a hot, humid environment). You do need to be careful with salt tablets, however; there are a number of them on the market, and almost all provide different amounts of sodium. I have seen some as low as 80 milligrams and some as high as 400 milligrams of sodium per tablet. Please see the table in the appendix (page 182) for a comparison of electrolyte or salt tablets available on the market today.

The amount of sodium you lose in your sweat is highly individual. On average, every liter of sweat contains approximately 1,000 milligrams of sodium (although the range is between 500 to 1,700 milligrams), and only about 150 to 200 milligrams of potassium. That means if you sweat at a rate of 1 liter per hour for a five-hour half Ironman race, then you may lose approximately 5,000 milligrams (although the range can be between 2,500 and 8,500 milligrams) of sodium for your entire race.

You may notice that this is a pretty wide range. This is because some people are salty sweaters and some are not. If you are a salty sweater (and you can tell if you are because you can actually see the salt accumulate on your clothes and skin) and/or you race in a hot, humid environment, then you probably need to be at the higher end of the recommendation in order to replace those losses. In general, I do not recommend that you consume more than 1,000 milligrams (or 1 gram) of sodium per hour. If you are a salty sweater, you may need up to 1 gram of sodium per hour. If you don't sweat a lot, or don't think that you lose much sodium in your sweat, then 0.5 grams (or 500 milligrams) per hour will probably work.

In general, triathletes should consume one to three tablets of a fairly high concentration of sodium during their race, along with products (such as gels and sports drinks) that contain sodium. Practice taking these during training sessions to help you determine what amount to use. Some triathletes have a hard time handling salt tablets; I know one who gets severe GI cramping anytime he takes one. Again, if you practice with these, then you will have discovered this fact during training sessions.

If you get cramping (muscle or GI) the first time you take a salt tablet, don't give up on them. Try it again, and make sure you drink a lot of water when you take the tablet. If you continue to have cramping, try taking a tablet that has lower amounts of sodium in it (such as 80mg). This amount, in conjunction with a lot of water, should prevent cramping from occurring. If for some reason you continue to get cramping, stop taking the tablets, because they can do more harm than good. Instead, focus on eating some foods that are rich in electrolytes, especially sodium.

Protein: You will use some protein for energy during a half Ironman race, but it won't be a major source. Therefore, protein should not be one of your main considerations during a race. There is some evidence that consuming small amounts of protein (specifically, branched-chain amino acids) can help with endurance performance. I don't think there's enough evidence to support this—yet—so if you want to take in some protein during your race, that's fine; it just shouldn't be a major focus. Some products (such as Accel Gels) contain a 4:1 ratio of carbs to protein, which means you will get some protein if you consume this hourly. I also know that eating protein can help prevent "flavor fatigue," which is feeling nauseous or sick at the thought of consuming certain foods or beverages. Flavor fatigue commonly occurs when you have to eat a certain flavor too often and get "sick" of it. This usually happens with carbohydrates, or, more important, sugars, during long bouts of exercise (we will talk about this more in chapters 10 and 14). If that works for you, do it on race day, too. Just remember that your focus should be on getting the adequate amount of carbohydrates.

Fat: I recommend eating no fat during a Sprint or Olympic distance triathlon because those are high-intensity races. While you may be doing your half Ironman at a high intensity as well, it is usually not quite as intense as it would be for those shorter-distance races. Generally, triathletes can handle dietary fat better if they exercise at lower intensities. Some athletes also get tired of only taking in carbohydrates for a three-hour bike ride and a two-hour run. (I know; some of you are faster and some slower—this is just a middle ground.)

I have seen triathletes eat PB&J sandwiches, Snickers bars, and Combos snacks during their bike ride. All of these have fat in them (some more than others). The biggest drawback of fat consumption during racing is the possibility of GI distress. Therefore, if you can handle some fat during racing, by all means, go ahead. Dietary fat will slow down digestion and absorption of other nutrients (carbohydrates and protein), though, so don't consume too much, because you need to be getting those carbs into the bloodstream on a regular basis.

Post-Race Nutrition

Congratulations! You have finished a half Ironman race. Whether it was your first one or your fiftieth, it's a great accomplishment. Don't celebrate too soon, however; make sure you get your post-race nutrition in, and then you can celebrate to your heart's content. Guess what you need to focus on for your post-race nutrition? Yup, that's right: carbohydrates and fluids, along with protein. Try to consume this first meal within that critical fifteen to thirty minutes after finishing. There will probably be a food tent where you can get some things to eat and drink after your race. However, these are usually carbohydrate-rich and do not contain much (if any) protein. Therefore, do not depend on the race director to provide the nutrients that you need after the race. Instead, bring your own recovery meal. Liquid calories are an excellent choice for this post-race meal because you probably won't feel like eating a steak dinner right after racing. (If you do, then I don't think you raced hard enough; either that, or you're a superstar!)

Carbohydrates: Consume 1.2 grams of carbohydrate per kilogram of body weight. Here is how you can calculate your own carbohydrate needs:

1. Your weight (in kilograms): _____ x 1.2 grams = _____ grams of carbohydrate.

2. Since there are 4 calories for each gram of carbohydrate, this equates to _____ calories of carbohydrate (your gram number x 4).

CALCULATING POST-RACE CARBOHYDRATE INTAKE: An Example

This triathlete weighs 80 kilograms (176 pounds).

1. 80 kilograms x 1.2 grams of carbohydrate = 96 grams of carbohydrate.
2. Since there are 4 calories per gram of carbohydrate, this meal will contain 384 calories of carbohydrate (96 grams x 4 calories per gram = 384 calories).

The type of carbohydrates in this post-race meal should have a high glycemic index (high in sugars). This allows for rapid digestion and absorption so you can start replenishing your glycogen stores as quickly as possible.

This recommendation of 1.2 grams of carbohydrate per kilogram of body weight should be consumed within fifteen to thirty minutes, and then again each hour for the next two to three hours. This will help to ensure complete glycogen repletion. If you eat right after the race but then don't eat for the next several hours, you will not recover adequately. This is especially true for a race of this distance, or any longer races.

Protein: You do need protein in your post-race meal, but not much. Shoot for 6 to 20 grams of protein (24 to 80 calories) from a complete protein source (contains all nine essential amino acids). Remember that protein is needed right after racing for the repair and rebuilding of body tissues, but this building process will stop if you are missing an essential amino acid that is needed for a particular body protein. This is why you need complete protein sources. Remember, soy and all animal proteins are complete proteins. If you consume plant proteins (other than soy), then just make sure you combine different plant sources so you will get all nine essential amino acids. If you go over 20 grams, that is fine. However, getting more than 20 grams does not enhance protein synthesis, repair, or recovery any more than 20 grams of complete protein.

Make Note: Six to 20 grams of protein from a complete protein source (any animal protein and soy, since they contain all nine essential amino acids) should be consumed within fifteen to thirty minutes after racing to repair and rebuild body tissues.

Fat: You don't have to worry about dietary fat causing GI problems. However, it does slow down digestion and absorption, so for your first post-race meal, try not to load up on dietary fat. It's important to get carbohydrates and proteins into the body as quickly as possible, and fat will only slow that down. Therefore, try to keep fat low in this first meal. There are a number of recovery drinks available on the market. Personally, I am a huge fan of low-fat chocolate milk. In fact, research has actually shown that chocolate milk promotes recovery to the same extent as, or possibly even better than, some commercially available recovery drinks. Chocolate milk has a decent amount of carbohydrates (many of which are sugars), adequate amounts of protein, and is low in fat (assuming you choose the low-fat option).

Fluids: Even if you followed your hydration plan and recommendations during your race, you will likely be a little dehydrated when you finish. Begin the rehydration process as soon as you can. If you have a scale around, then you can use pre- and post-race body weights to determine fluid loss. (Sorry; you didn't lose 3 pounds of fat during your race—it's almost all water weight.) Drink 1 to 2 cups of fluid for every pound lost. Drink this amount gradually over a couple of hours; do not drink really large amounts at one time because it can dilute blood sodium levels and cause hyponatremia. Alternatively, you can drink some water and some sports drinks that have electrolytes in them. If you do not have a scale available (which is the most likely scenario), drink until your urine is a pale yellow color and urination occurs once every one to two hours.

Vitamins and Minerals: During your race, you have lost electrolytes, used some B vitamins (since they assist with energy production), and used some antioxidants as well. If you eat a variety of fruits and vegetables throughout the day following your race, as well as a salty meal or two, you will replenish those micronutrients. Additionally, if you take a daily multi-vitamin/mineral pill, take it after your race to replace some of the nutrients that were lost during the race. That being said, there is no need to take mega-doses of any particular vitamin or mineral. People often do this with anti-oxidants (such as vitamin C or vitamin E) and B vitamins. Vitamin C and your B vitamins are water-soluble, so any extra that your body can't use will be excreted in the urine (so you're just making expensive urine). If you eat a balanced diet for the remainder of the day after your race, you will be just fine. So, save your money for something more important than high doses of a micronutrient.

CHAPTER 10

Full Ironman Triathlon

The Ironman is the granddaddy of all triathlons. Whether you are a first-time Ironman competitor or a seasoned veteran, the Ironman race is special. You most likely have spent (or will spend) months training for this race and have sacrificed a great deal of your free time in order to spend it in the pool, on the bike, or pounding the pavement. I saved this chapter for last in this section of the book because nutrition for this race is more important than for any other race. Small nutrition mistakes here can equate to hours added to your overall finish, or a dreaded DNF (did not finish). Likewise, you need to plan your race-day nutrition more carefully for this race than for any other. If this is your first Ironman, then you have the chance to get your nutrition right on the first try, thanks to this book. If you are a previous Ironman finisher, here's an opportunity to actually make a formal nutrition plan for race day and avoid those mistakes you've made in previous races.

When I work with Ironman triathletes, I always assume they have a pretty good handle on what nutrients they need during a race. However, this is not always the case. I often ask triathletes how many carbohydrates they plan to eat per hour during their race. Their answers vary from "about 300 calories" (calories are not the answer to this question—it's about carbohydrates), to "I don't know the actual amount, but I eat two gels an hour," to "I'm not really sure—I just go by feel and when I think I need some calories or energy." As you can see, it is common for these athletes to overlook their nutrition, which is a huge mistake. If you can develop a great nutrition plan, think of the advantage you will have over all those Ironman competitors who haven't come as prepared.

In addition to the breakdown of meals that I review in my other chapters, I also include some helpful hints in this chapter on how to avoid flavor fatigue, what "liquid gold" is, and how to combat a surly stomach on race day.

Twenty-Four Hours Before the Race

For many triathletes (especially first-time Ironman racers), nerves can really ramp up the day before the race. There is also plenty of hustle and bustle before an Ironman race. Keep in mind that you have a long day ahead of you, so take it easy and get some relaxation before your race. It's also important to make sure you eat adequate amounts of food and drink sufficient liquids the day before your big race. You should not feel hungry the day before the race; if you do, make sure you eat something right away. Always carry water around with you everywhere you go, and be sure to drink it throughout the day. The biggest mistake you could make would be to miss a meal or be slightly dehydrated that close to the race.

I also recommend staying out of the sun. I recently did Ironman Canada, and there's a really nice beach where the swim start is. I saw tons of triathletes lying out in the sun, building sand castles with their kids, and playing around in the lake. Now, I'm all for family fun, but don't risk sunburn or dehydration (or just fatigue from being in the sun all day) before your race. You can always crash on the beach and relax the day after your race (you will have earned it).

Just like all of the other races I've written about in this book, carbohydrates and fluids should be your primary focus. It's important to make sure your glycogen levels are topped off, so aim for 60 to 75 percent of total calories from carbohydrates. The 75 percent recommendation is higher than for any other race, which shows how important it is to make sure you get plenty of carbs. After you take care of your carbohydrate needs, 10 to 20 percent of calories should come from protein, and the remainder from fat (20 to 30 percent). If you get 75 percent of calories from carbohydrates, your fat intake for that day may be on the low side (around 15 percent); that's fine, since it's just one day of a low-fat diet. Fluid recommendations were covered in chapter 6; follow those to be sure you're well hydrated.

The same do's and don'ts for the other races apply for an Ironman race as well:

Summary of Nutrition Tips for 24-Hours Pre-Race

1. Do focus on complex carbohydrates, lean, complete protein sources (those that contain all nine essential amino acids, which are any animal product, soy, or combinations of plant proteins), and good sources of fat (rich in MUFAs and PUFAs).

2. Do remember to take your multivitamin/mineral pill so you get adequate amounts of all of your micronutrients.

3. Do make sure your dinner the evening before the race contains mostly carbohydrates, some lean protein, and just a little fat.

4. Do not eat a lot of fiber the day before the race, especially at your evening meal. Cut back on the fiber by about 30 to 50 percent. If you usually eat 25 grams of fiber each day, then aim for 12 to 17 grams. If you don't want to count up grams of fiber, then just try to cut back on or minimize whole grains, beans/legumes, and vegetables (for that day only).

Now, everyone has their "favorite" pre-race foods—I've heard of people eating an entire pizza and half a pan of brownies—but in addition to cutting back on fiber, I also recommend that you don't eat huge amounts of simple sugars, because you may wake up feeling sluggish. You will lose a lot of sodium when you sweat on race day, so make sure you eat some salty foods the day before your race. Again, though, I wouldn't recommend eating a ton of salt the evening before, because you may wake up feeling like you have a hangover, or, at the very least, you may feel quite bloated.

Most triathletes do not sleep very well the night before an Ironman, so if you find yourself waking up during the night, you may want to hydrate and refuel. Have a bottle of water by your bedside and drink a little if you wake up during the night. (Of course, this may cause you to wake up an hour or two later, needing to use the bathroom.) You may also want to have something easy to eat. I usually keep my favorite flavor of PowerBar nearby so that if I wake up, I can get some calories and carbohydrates in. There is logic behind this. If you remember from chapter 1, your liver is virtually depleted of glycogen after an overnight fast. Therefore, if you eat some during the night, you may not wake up as depleted of glycogen. This can be very helpful for triathletes who don't have much of an appetite on race morning.

Pre-Race Nutrition

Most Ironman races start at 7:00 a.m. That means you should probably be up by 4:00 a.m. so you will have two and a half to three hours to eat your pre-race meal. If you follow the upper end of the recommendation below, then you may need to get up a little earlier. You will need carbohydrates throughout the day, so it's important to get enough in your pre-race meal to top off glycogen stores and replenish what was lost during your overnight fast. The pre-race meal should be rich in carbohydrates, can contain some protein, and should have very little fat. For this distance race, aim for 2.0 to 3.5 grams of carbohydrate per kilogram of body weight.

Here is how you calculate your intake:

1. Lower end of the range: Your weight (in kilograms): _____
   x 2.0 grams = _____ grams of carbohydrate. Since there are 4 calories for each gram of carbohydrate, this equates to _____ calories of carbohydrate (your gram number x 4).

2. Upper end of the range: Your weight (in kilograms): _____
   x 3.5 grams = _____ grams of carbohydrate. Since there are 4 calories for each gram of carbohydrate, this equates to _____ calories of carbohydrate (your gram number x 4).

Remember to keep this meal low in fiber, and don't eat a lot of simple sugars within one hour of your race. There are some sample pre-race meals listed in the appendix.

Protein: You will use slightly more protein for energy for an Ironman than you will for any other triathlon. With a race of this length, your body may get up to 15 percent of energy from protein (usually, it is 5 to 10 percent). However, eating a lot of protein before you start your race probably won't help much with the protein you will use during racing. Any extra protein that you eat gets converted to fat and stored; you cannot store protein in

CALCULATING YOUR PRE-RACE CARBOHYDRATE INTAKE RANGE: An Example

This triathlete weighs 80 kilograms (176 pounds).

1. Lower end of range: 80 kilograms x 2.0 grams of carbohydrate = 160 grams of carbohydrate. Since there are 4 calories for each gram of carbohydrate, this equates to 640 calories (160 grams x 4 calories per gram = 640 calories).
2. Upper end of range: 80 kilograms x 3.5 grams of carbohydrate = 280 grams of carbohydrate. Since there are 4 calories for each gram of carbohydrate, this equates to 1,120 calories (280 grams x 4 calories per gram = 1,120 calories). Therefore, the total carbohydrate calories for this meal range from 640 to 1,120 calories.

the body to use it for energy later in the day. So, small amounts of protein are good, but focus on carbohydrates.

Fat: Just like with any other race, you want to keep fat intake fairly low. Some triathletes eat more fat before an Ironman race compared to a Sprint because they plan on racing at a lower intensity for the Ironman race. Whatever your personal preference, make sure you have plenty of time to allow the fat you eat to be fully digested and absorbed (so, this means no fat intake within two hours of the race start). It can be quite difficult to eat a pre-race meal without any fat, so as long as you've practiced taking in fat, you should be fine on race day. In your pre-race meal, try not to go above 15 percent of calories from fat.

Fluids: Fluid intake is extremely important on race morning. If you wake up three to four hours before your race, drink 1 to 2 cups as soon as possible. Then drink another cup two hours before the race, and one final cup of fluid about thirty minutes before the race. Water is an excellent choice, but you can drink other fluids if it is two to four hours before the race (especially if you need the carbohydrates to make up part of your pre-race meal). However, once you get to one hour before the race, you should stick to water for any fluid intake (you don't want a lot of sugar that close to the race). As I've mentioned previously, many triathletes drink coffee on a daily basis. If this is you, then make sure you also drink it on race morning. It is a diuretic (which can cause water loss), but as long as you drink water and don't make your coffee too strong, you will not lose more fluids than you take in.

One last thing that I'll mention about this pre-race meal has to do with nerves and appetite. Most triathletes are nervous before an Ironman, especially for the first one. You need to find a way to calm down enough to eat breakfast. A friend of mine always ate cereal and milk before training sessions. So, on race morning of his first Ironman, he poured himself a big bowl of cereal and milk and dove in. He got one bite into it before he turned green and broke out in a cold sweat. He couldn't even swallow that first bite. If you are as nervous as my friend was, try a liquid breakfast. Liquid calories are usually easier to get down than solid food when you have butterflies. I include a liquid meal option in the appendix along with some other pre-race meals.

Make Note: If you get really nervous before a race, consider a liquid pre-race meal. Liquid meals are usually easier than solid foods to "get down" when you have pre-race jitters. Whatever you do, do not skip this meal!

During-Race Nutrition

If you do an Ironman distance race, hopefully you have practiced your nutrition on all those long training rides and runs. Any experienced Ironman athlete knows that it's a long day and a lot can happen (and go wrong), even with the best nutrition plans. You should write out your race nutrition plan ahead of time and memorize it. I say this because many triathletes start racing and seem to forget that they even had a nutrition plan, much less actually follow it. I've competed in and volunteered for enough Ironman events to see just about everything. Some athletes seem to completely lose their heads once the gun goes off. This is not a good thing. You want to remain calm, cool, and collected during your race. That is the only way you will be able to pull off your race (including your nutrition plans) successfully.

Throughout this section, we will focus on the Big Three: carbohydrates, fluids, and electrolytes. In addition to that, I will provide some tips and pointers for other problems you may encounter during an Ironman race and what you can do to prevent or minimize those problems.

> **Make Note:** The longer the race distance, the more important it is to focus your nutrition around the Big Three: carbohydrates, fluids, and electrolytes.

Carbohydrates: Since an Ironman race is several hours long, you should aim for the higher end of the carbohydrate recommendation. For shorter races, 60 to 70 grams of carbohydrate per hour is the recommendation; for an Ironman race, 60 to 90 grams of carbohydrate per hour is best. If you can tolerate 90 grams per hour, then by all means, consume that amount. Many athletes can't handle that much for that long, though, so make sure you are getting at least 60 grams per hour, and see if you can handle slightly higher amounts for a few hours.

Remember that you can practice and train your body to tolerate slightly higher amounts of carbs. If you started out being able to consume 60 grams per hour, maybe by the end of the season (and on race day), you will be able to consume about 70 to 80 grams per hour. You want a mixture of glucose and fructose, which you will get from all sports drinks and sports-nutrition products. Stay away from a lot of complex carbohydrates (as they take too long to digest and absorb) and fiber. High-glycemic-index (high-sugar) foods are your best bet.

Fluids: Getting enough fluids in during an Ironman race is more important than in any other distance race. You can still finish a Sprint, Olympic, or even half Ironman distance race when you are dehydrated, but if you don't consume enough fluids during an Ironman race, you will be very lucky to make it to the finish line. Since you won't be able to drink during the swim (at least not intentionally), make sure you start drinking fluids as soon as you get on the bike.

You should perform sweat trials during biking and running sessions (see chapter 6 for a review), so you can determine your fluid needs and try to match them. For example, if you need an average of 3.7 cups per hour, then drink about 4 cups per hour. As I've mentioned before, the math doesn't always work out. Some athletes have really high sweat rates and simply cannot replace fluids quickly enough to match losses. Most triathletes can absorb about 1 liter (4.2 cups) of fluid while biking and slightly less while running (maybe only about half to three-quarters of a liter (~2 to 3 cups). Therefore, if you need 7 cups per hour based on your sweat rate, you will slowly dehydrate over the course of the day.

All you can do to try to minimize dehydration is to drink as much as possible. In training, you should have started out with 4 cups per hour on the bike and then gradually increased that amount to see what you could tolerate. The same applies for running (only starting at about 2 to 3 cups per hour and working your way up from there). If you haven't done a sweat trial, then the recommendation is 1 cup every ten to twenty minutes. I recommend getting a mixture of water and sports drinks for your fluid intake. The water is good to help wash down the food you eat and helps prevent flavor fatigue, while the sports drinks are good for providing electrolytes and carbohydrates.

Make Note: Use your calculated sweat rate to determine fluid needs. If you haven't performed a sweat trial, then try to drink 1 cup every ten to twenty minutes.

Electrolytes: For electrolytes, you are primarily concerned with sodium. You will also lose potassium and chloride (and some other electrolytes) through sweat, but sodium losses will be the greatest. Sweat generally contains approximately 1,000 milligrams of sodium, but the range for people can be between 500 to 1,700 milligrams of sodium per liter of sweat. A sweat rate of 1 liter per hour for a twelve-hour race would therefore cause a salt loss of approximately 12,000 milligrams (or 12 grams) of sodium, although the range may be between 6,000 to 20,000 milligrams (6 to 20 grams). Failing to replace salt during the race will certainly diminish performance, but it can also result in hyponatremia.

It is important for Ironman athletes to replace electrolytes just as they replace fluid losses. Sports drinks and sports-nutrition products almost always contain electrolytes. However, those products and drinks are usually not enough to replace the amount that you lose through sweat. That is where electrolyte or salt tablets come into play. In general, an athlete doing an Ironman race should aim for up to 1 gram (1,000 milligrams) of sodium per hour, especially in a hot and humid environment. Again, it is important to practice this during training sessions so you will know how your body tolerates this level of salt. I provide a list of electrolyte tablet products in the appendix. Each brand of electrolytes contains different amounts of sodium, so read the label carefully. If you get about 500 milligrams of sodium an hour from food/drink products, then you need only about 300 to 500 milligrams more from salt tablets. This means taking one salt tablet from certain products, and three to five tablets from other products. It is also important to drink plenty of fluids (especially water) when you take a salt tablet. If you don't, you're setting yourself up for some serious GI or muscle cramping.

Make Note: Each brand of electrolyte or salt tablet can contain very different amounts of sodium. Make sure you read the label carefully when planning your intake.

Fats and Proteins: You don't want to eat a lot of fat or protein during the race because both nutrients can cause some GI complications. In general, protein is tolerated much better than fat. Additionally, there is some research to support small amounts of protein intake during long-duration exercise. This protein can be used as an energy source. There is no recommended amount of protein intake during racing; however, you shouldn't consume more than 20 grams an hour, because if you do, you are likely neglecting your carbohydrate needs.

As far as dietary fat is concerned, this comes down more to personal preference than anything else. If you can tolerate some fat during racing, then go ahead (especially if it helps with flavor fatigue, which I will discuss later in this section). However, keep in mind that fat will delay digestion and absorption, which is not a good thing when it comes to getting a steady supply of carbohydrates into the bloodstream, and it can also cause GI distress. If you're already not feeling well on race day, then stay away from those foods or snacks with modest to high amounts of fat in them.

Swim Portion of Race

In addition to focusing on carbohydrates, fluids, and electrolytes, you also need to remember this slogan: Early and often. What does this mean? Since the race is so long, you want to preserve your glycogen stores and prevent dehydration for as long as you can. This means consuming food and fluids soon after the start of the race, and continuing to do so throughout the day. This poses the first problem with your race-day nutrition plan—the swim. I have seen triathletes tuck gels into their wetsuits, so I'm assuming that some of them actually eat during the swim. The swim portion can get a little physical (yes, that's a drastic understatement), so for practical reasons, don't count on taking in any food or fluids during this part of the race. For you speed demons out there, this means that, within one hour of starting, you will be able to eat. However, for others, it may be about ninety minutes to two hours before you can eat or drink anything.

Bike Portion of Race

If you're not worried about your overall time, then eat a gel and drink some water in transition. However, if you want to spend as little time as possible in transition, then eat and drink something within the first two miles of your bike ride. I recommend a gel and some water because it is easy to get down and people are usually slightly out of breath and have a slightly elevated heart rate from transition. It usually takes a couple of miles on the bike to settle into your target pace.

From that initial time that you eat, you should think of eating every twenty to thirty minutes and drinking more frequently than that. A good friend of mine is terrible at remembering to eat or drink, so she sets a timer on her watch to go off every ten minutes. That means, every ten minutes she drinks and/or eats something. Now, you need to have all of this planned out ahead of time, because after a couple of hours, it can be easy to forget when you last ate and what you're supposed to eat next. Imagine how hard it would be to keep track of everything if you hadn't ever written anything down or tried to memorize it.

You should also look at the course map (if you haven't biked or run on the course) ahead of time and plan your eating schedule accordingly. For example, if you have an 11-kilometer mountain to climb up at mile 40 (such as Richter Pass at Ironman Canada), you probably want to plan your nutrition around that. If you don't plan for the route, then you may get halfway up the mountain and realize that you are now supposed to eat a PB&J sandwich. Most likely, that won't work. So, plan your food and fluid intake in accordance with the course as much as possible.

For an Ironman race, you will probably take most of your food with you on the bike. Some triathletes rely solely on the aid stations, but most athletes carry their favorite foods with them. You should know what mile (and approximate hour) you will get to your bike special needs bag (a bag you fill prior to the race with anything and everything you want to have available about halfway through the bike portion of the race). If you take all of your food with you, make sure you pack an extra gel or two. You may find that you're having a rough day and fall behind your planned schedule. If that is the case, at least you know that you have enough food to get you to the next aid station.

Make Note: When planning your food and fluid intake for the bike portion, consider these things carefully: 1) At what mile markers will you find the aid stations? 2) What will the aid stations provide? 3) Are there technical or difficult parts of the course where food/fluid intake may not be feasible?

Another thing to keep in mind for an Ironman race is the size of your fluid bottles. You may train with a few favorite bottles, meaning you know exactly how much fluid they hold so it's easy to keep track of your intake. During the race, you will probably get some fluids from the aid stations. Pay attention to the bottle sizes (16 ounces versus 20 and 24 ounces) so you know how many cups are in each.

Triathletes also run into problems when they pour fluids into their aerodynamic fluid holders on their bikes. If you drink out of something like that, it can be rather difficult to keep track of your fluid intake. I recommend that you drink every ten minutes to make sure you empty the containers in a reasonable time based on their size. For example, if your aerodynamic container holds 32 ounces (4 cups), then you should drink it all in about an hour.

Finally, the last problem triathletes run into with keeping track of fluid intake is tracking the fluids that get thrown out. I see quite a few athletes dumping their mostly empty bottles out right before the aid station to get a fresh bottle of water or sports drink. This is fine, except it's important to remember that you didn't drink all of the contents of that bottle. You may think you've consumed seven bottles of fluid on the bike, but if you threw out 25 percent of each of those bottles, then you didn't get nearly as much as you thought.

I am providing all of this information not to overwhelm you, but rather to give you an idea of how complicated it can be to both plan and execute proper race-day nutrition. The most successful triathletes can execute their nutrition plan and adapt to roadblocks or problems that arise. Some of this comes from experience, but a lot of it is simply smart planning; that's why you really need to write out your nutrition plan ahead of time and follow all of the tips in this chapter.

Run Portion of Race

For as many complications as there are on the bike, there are just as many on the run. During training, you probably used some type of fuel belt and drank out of those bottles. When you get to the run portion of an Ironman, you will be handed cups that have varying amounts of fluids in them. This poses two problems: First, you don't know how much fluid is in each of those cups (volunteers simply pour a certain amount into each cup, so they all vary). Second, it's not as easy as it may seem to drink water from a cup while running. For every 4 ounces of fluid in the cup, you may only get 2 to 3 ounces in your mouth (and the rest runs down the front of your shirt). If you walk through aid stations, however, then the second problem becomes a nonissue.

If you are really worried about getting in enough fluids and food on the run, then it may be a good idea to walk through those aid stations. However, if you're trying to PR (attain a personal record) or compete in your age group, then you need to be able to eat and drink while running. So, if you spill some fluids and each cup has a different amount, how do you know how much to take? The answer is . . . I don't know. For this reason, some athletes choose to wear a fuel belt while racing and refill or replace their bottles. I personally don't like racing with a belt, so I pay close attention to what I drink and try to consume fluids at every aid station. You can also put a crease in your cup while running, which helps to reduce the amount of fluid that spills out when you drink. In general, it's a good idea to try to drink something at every aid station.

Another problem that you may encounter during the marathon is that you have to rely on aid stations for some food. I personally consume only gels during the marathon (unless I'm experiencing nausea, and then I try whatever I can get to work). However, I can't carry enough gels on me to get me to my run special needs bag (a bag you fill prior to the race with anything and everything you want to have available about half-way through the run portion of the race). That means I end up eating a gel or two on the course. You're probably thinking, What's the big deal? Well, each brand of gel tastes quite different, so hopefully you can find a brand that you like. The other problem is the flavor (not to be mistaken with flavor fatigue).

I can vividly recall a problem that I had with flavor during my second Ironman Wisconsin. I was at about mile 12 and needed to take a gel. The only flavor available at the aid station was mocha. For most people, this wouldn't be a problem. However, I strongly dislike coffee—even the smell of it is repulsive to me. So, imagine my dismay when I realized I was going to have to eat a mocha-flavored gel. I literally choked it down because I knew it was more important to get those carbs in than to wait until I reached my special needs bag. Therefore, you not only have to worry about flavor fatigue, but the actual flavors or types of products that are available on the course and whether you like them enough to eat them.

If your stomach is already a little upset, the wrong-flavored gel can be enough to push you over the edge. I recommend carrying as many of your own products as you can and then hoping for the best while on the course. Remember: Don't skip eating just because you don't like the flavor. It's better to eat something you don't like than to miss out on the calories altogether.

Complications with Nutrition

For many different reasons, the majority of triathletes get some GI distress (nausea, cramping, and diarrhea) during an Ironman race. If you tend to get sharp stomach pains or cramping, it's a good guess that it's the result of dehydration and/or electrolyte imbalance. If this happens, try to take in some fluids (sports drinks are preferred here because they have both water and electrolytes). If you can't take in fluids, then you will have to wait it out. You may have to slow down or stop completely until you're able to get some type of liquid in.

If you get stomach cramping, I wouldn't recommend taking a salt or electrolyte tablet unless you can drink large amounts of water with it. Athletes with cramping often can't drink fluids, so taking a salt tablet without fluid will only make the problem worse. For those athletes who experience nausea and/or diarrhea (which seems to be more common than cramping), the following paragraphs provide some helpful hints and suggestions for things to try.

Flavor fatigue is another real problem during an Ironman race. You may get to the point where you would rather not eat than have to eat another gel. I have a few suggestions for preventing or minimizing flavor fatigue. First, don't eat the same thing all day long. I personally like to eat more foods that have to be chewed on the bike (because it's easier to eat while biking) and save gels for the run. For example, I eat a lot of Clif Shot Bloks on the bike and then all gels on the run. I also mix up the flavors of the gels or other products so I'm getting some variety.

One of the best things for curing flavor fatigue is some salt. I don't mean taking a salt tablet. You actually have to eat some salty food (which doesn't include a sweet taste). I usually eat a package of crackers with cheese in them at about mile 70 or 80 on the bike, when I'm starting to get sick of sweet-tasting food. Other things that work well are Combos, potato chips, and beef jerky. Some of these things are hard to eat, but if you start to feel nauseous or have severe flavor fatigue, slow down a little and eat some of this stuff. Of course, make sure you practice with these things during training sessions so you know you can tolerate them on race day.

When you get to the run, aid stations usually have pretzels and chicken broth. The chicken broth is a great choice for flavor fatigue and an upset stomach. It's easy to swallow and may just save your day. If salty foods don't help with your nausea, then try some other things. Protein is another nutrient that can help prevent flavor fatigue (that's why so many people like beef or turkey jerky—it has both salt and meat flavor). Other people swear by flat cola on the run (it's often referred to as liquid gold, because it really calms the stomachs of many triathletes). Fruit and other solid foods may also work. I have a friend who swears by mini Snickers when she starts to feel sick. The point is that you should try eating different things during practice (especially the foods/fluids that will be available at aid stations); that way, you can consume these different things on race day and they won't seem foreign to your stomach.

The last thing that I can recommend for calming your stomach during the race is Pepto-Bismol chewables. These saved me during my second Ironman, and I know many other triathletes who swear by them as well. If you get some really serious GI problems on race day, try a chewable or two. It may be the thing that saves your race, too.

> **Make Note:** Many Ironman athletes experience GI problems on race day. Some stomach savers to try include salty foods such as beef jerky, crackers, or chicken broth, flat cola on the run, fruit or other citrus/refreshing foods, and Pepto-Bismol chewables.

I never recommend trying anything new on race day that you haven't done in training. The one exception to that is if you get sick and your nutrition plan simply isn't working. If that's the case, then try anything and everything. If you're sick and unable to eat, you're already in a bad place. By trying different foods or drinks, you may just find the cure to get you to the finish line.

Many Ironman races now use a sports drink provided by the race sponsor. Unfortunately, these drinks are not often found in your regular supermarket. For example, some races use Gatorade Endurance Formula or PowerBar Ironman Perform. Both of these are next to impossible to find in a grocery store. I recommend purchasing some over the Internet so you can practice with the product before the race; that way there won't be any surprises on race day. The same goes for the food products that are provided at the race. If you only use Accel Gels and have to eat Gu Gels on race day, your body won't be used to them. So, buy some gels or other foods that will be available on the course.

Despite all this talk about the things that could go wrong, it's important to note that not every triathlete experiences these issues. On any given day, a triathlete can feel great and not experience any of these problems; however, it's more than likely that at some point during the race, you will not feel entirely well. If you have a good nutrition plan and follow it during training sessions, you will be prepared if any such issues arise on race day, and you'll know how to deal with them.

Post-Race Nutrition

At the finish line of most Ironman races you will find pizza, cookies and donuts, pretzels, fruit, carbonated beverages, sports drinks, and water. The pizza always seems to be the most popular item. I think it's the saltiness that just tastes so good after a full day of eating sweet food. That first piece always tastes great—but a second piece is probably a mistake. Instead, eat one piece and then work on getting some lower-fat items that are rich in carbohydrates and protein into your system. If you don't have much of an appetite right after the race, try liquid calories. I usually keep a can of Boost or Ensure in my morning drop bag (the bag you have with you that you can put your warm-up clothes into before the start of the race) so that when I pick up all my bags (morning drop bag and transition bags) after the race, I can drink that if I don't feel like eating. For recovery, you want to focus on carbohydrates, protein, and fluids.

Carbohydrates: The recommendation is to consume 1.2 grams of carbohydrate per kilogram of body weight. This should be done within the first thirty minutes post-race. It should also be done for each subsequent hour over the next three to four hours. It sounds like a lot of food, but your body needs it. If you don't want to eat every hour, then get that first post-race meal in and then eat an even larger meal about two hours post-race. Ideal recovery, though, is to eat 1.2 grams of carbohydrates per kilogram of body weight hourly after a race of this distance, for about three to four hours, at least.

Here is how to calculate your own carbohydrate needs:

Your weight (in kilograms): _____ x 1.2 grams = _____ grams of carbohydrate. This equates to _____ calories of carbohydrate (your gram number x 4).

The type of carbohydrates in this post-race meal should have a high glycemic index (high in sugars). This allows for rapid digestion and absorption so you can start replenishing your glycogen stores as quickly as possible. Again, if you have a hard time eating right after the race, stick to liquid calories.

Protein: Although protein intake was not nearly as important before or during your Ironman, it is extremely important after the race. Your body

---

CALCULATING YOUR OWN POST-RACE CARBOHYDRATE NEEDS: An Example

This triathlete weighs 80 kilograms (176 pounds).

1. 80 kilograms x 1.2 grams of carbohydrate = 96 grams of carbohydrate.
2. There are 4 calories per gram of carbohydrate, so this meal will contain 384 calories of carbohydrate (96 grams x 4 calories per gram = 384 calories).

---

needs protein for rebuilding and repairing muscle tissue, and for making other proteins that your body needs to assist with recovery. The key is to get complete proteins (meaning they contain all nine essential amino acids). Complete proteins come from any animal protein, soy protein, or combinations of plant proteins. If your body is missing an essential amino acid and it needs that amino acid for building a new protein, protein synthesis will stop. Therefore, it is crucial that you eat the right types of dietary protein.

You don't need a whole lot of protein to get the recovery process going. Six to 20 grams of complete protein will get the job done. Consume that amount with your first post-race meal, and then again with each meal that you eat hourly for the first three to four hours post-race. Lean sources of protein are also preferred, because fat will slow down digestion and absorption of both the protein and the carbohydrates you eat. One last note about protein: You may need slightly greater amounts than normal in the first several days after the race. Your body needs time to recover, so extra protein will be needed during that large, initial recovery process.

Fat: Even though you have burned a huge number of calories, many of which were fat calories, dietary fat is still not a priority for the post-race period. As I've mentioned in previous chapters, dietary fat will slow down digestion and absorption of other important nutrients. Therefore, keep fat intake low for the first one or two post-race meals. If you can't resist the post-race pizza and cookies that are served, remember to eat just one piece of pizza and one or two cookies, and make sure you also eat plenty of other carbohydrates and proteins. After you have consumed your important nutrients in the first and second hours post-race, you can increase the fat intake in the rest of your meals for the day. By then, the delay in delivery of carbohydrates and proteins into the bloodstream will not likely inhibit your recovery very much.

> **Make Note:** Keep fat intake to a minimum during your first post-race meal. Fat will only slow down digestion and absorption of carbohydrates and proteins, both of which are needed immediately to begin the recovery process.

Fluids: The fluid recommendations do not change much from those of a half Ironman race. The only difference is that you will probably be more dehydrated, so 100 percent rehydration will likely take a longer period of time. The most important thing is to start rehydrating as soon as possible after the race. You may not be fully rehydrated by the time you go to bed after an Ironman, so continue drinking fluids throughout the next day (or two) after the race. Again, water and sports drinks are excellent choices. If there is a scale available (nearly all Ironman medical tents have a scale), weigh yourself after the race and rehydrate accordingly (2 to 3 cups of fluid for each pound lost). Again, it may actually take a day or two to accomplish full rehydration. Do not drink huge amounts of water at one time, as this can dilute blood sodium levels too much and risk causing hyponatremia. If you don't have the option to weigh yourself right after the race, drink fluids hourly for the rest of the night, and then continue to drink fluids the following day until your urine is a pale yellow color and you urinate every one to two hours.

Vitamins and Minerals: For a race of this distance, you will likely have used extra amounts of B vitamins, antioxidants, and electrolytes. Eat salty foods to replace electrolytes, and fruits and vegetables to replace antioxidants and B vitamins. (B vitamins are found in many foods, including fruits, vegetables, whole grains, nuts, legumes, dairy products, and meats.) Additionally, take a multivitamin/mineral pill after the race. This should help to replenish some of the nutrients lost. Continue to follow this healthy diet in the several days following the race to ensure that you provide your body with enough micronutrients to replenish those lost and to assist with the recovery process.

Part Three:
Special Topics

At this point, you have the knowledge and tools not only to eat a healthy diet on a daily basis, but also to optimize your training and racing nutrition plans. You might be surprised to learn that the questions I get asked most often are about some of the issues and topics we haven't even covered yet. (I know— how could there possibly be more?) Part three of this book is designed to provide answers to those common issues that every triathlete seems to experience at one time or another.

The most recurring questions are regarding travel, illness, weight loss, nutritional supplements, and preventing GI distress during a race. I think these questions are asked so frequently because problems in any one of these areas can ruin a race, or in some cases, prevent you from even starting a race. At the very least, these issues may decrease your performance potential. After reading these chapters, some or all of your questions about these various topics should be answered. You can't always control things like illness or injury, but now you will have the nutrition tools to help you deal with a number of situations you may find yourself in.

CHAPTER 11

Weight Loss and Weight Maintenance

Most triathletes are very conscious of their body weight and usually have a vested interest in weight loss or weight maintenance. This is surprising to a lot of people, particularly those who are just getting into the sport of triathlon. Every time I go to a race venue, I feel like I'm surrounded by completely buff, ripped, lean athletes—and those are just the females. This is often an intimidating environment for first-time or recreational triathletes. It may come as a surprise to many people, but most triathletes battle their weight, including professional and competitive age-group triathletes. So this chapter will be centered on weight loss and weight maintenance. Very few triathletes are looking to gain weight, and those who do usually just want to put on a few pounds of muscle mass, which they can do by incorporating some strength training into their workout regime and eating an excess of about 300 to 500 calories per day.

Most people are aware that, in general, the lighter you are, the faster you can go. This is especially true for running (although it doesn't apply much for swimming). It is estimated that for every pound of weight lost, you can run anywhere from one to three seconds faster per mile. That may not seem like a lot (and maybe it doesn't matter at all if you're just looking to cross the finish line), but for those looking to PR or be competitive in their age group, a few seconds per mile can make a significant difference. A simple 5-pound weight loss can enable an athlete to finish fifteen to forty-five seconds faster for a Sprint triathlon (assuming a 5K run), and as much as two to six minutes faster for an Ironman race.

You may remember from the introduction to this book that the food you eat contains energy in the form of calories. When this energy is used by the body, we say it is expended energy, and we also measure this in calories. Changes in body weight all come down to one basic equation. It is called the energy balance equation. You can think of the energy balance equation as a balance scale. On one side of the equation you have energy intake (food intake measured in calories) and on the other side you have energy expenditure (also measured in calories). If energy intake matches energy expenditure, then the person is in energy balance, and body weight will not change. If a person is in a positive energy balance (energy intake is greater than energy expenditure), then weight gain will occur. Similarly, if a person is in a negative energy balance (energy intake is less than energy expenditure), then weight loss will occur.

> **Make Note:** Changes in body weight all boil down to the energy balance equation. If you consume more energy (calories) than you expend or burn, you will gain weight. If you consume less energy (calories) than you expend or burn, you will lose weight.

This equation seems simple enough, but actually achieving that negative energy balance is harder than it sounds (or maybe you already know that). Most people who lose weight do so by decreasing their total calories consumed through food and increasing their calories burned by exercising. However, if you are a triathlete, you are already exercising. If you exercise on a daily basis (or close to daily) and have been doing so for a while, you probably aren't losing weight on a weekly basis. Why is this? Well, your body is really good at knowing how much energy you expend. Therefore, when people increase their volume of exercise and burn more calories, they usually feel hungrier. Their body tries to replace those extra calories burned by taking in more food calories. This is the challenge that triathletes face. Although many triathletes have a very high caloric expenditure, they find that they also eat a lot more than their friends who don't exercise at all, because they feel hungrier.

The biggest challenge faced by triathletes who want to lose weight is finding a balance between their caloric (energy) deficit while still being able to maintain optimum training or performance levels. The number-one complaint by people who lose weight is a decrease in energy levels. Simply stated, they just feel tired. So, how does one go about losing weight (and if you do it right, losing body fat, not muscle) while still maintaining enough energy to train and stick with the diet? Let's break down weight loss by the numbers:

> **Make Note:** To lose 1 pound of fat, you need to have an energy (caloric) deficit of about 3,500 calories.

In order to lose 1 pound of fat, you need to have a caloric or energy deficit of 3,500 calories. You can achieve this by either increasing your energy expenditure by 3,500 calories, decreasing food/energy intake by 3,500 calories, or doing a combination of decreased food intake and increased energy expenditure. Just to give you an idea of how much exercise it takes to burn 3,500 calories, the table on the following page shows the energy cost of some activities (shown as calories expended during one hour of activity):

When you realize that a 155-pound person will only burn about 3,000 calories during an entire marathon, you begin to realize just how much exercise it takes to burn a pound of fat. When people ask me how to best go about losing weight, I usually recommend a combination of increasing the current exercise volume and decreasing food intake slightly. However, many triathletes do not want to exercise any more than they already do. I have two possible solutions for these athletes who want to lose weight: You will either have to do it all by decreasing food intake, or you can decrease food intake and slightly increase physical activity levels.

You may be a little confused about what I just said. Well, exercise and physical activity are not the same thing. When you train each day, you are performing exercise. Physical activity includes things like taking your dog for a walk, doing household chores, walking to/from your car, climbing stairs, etc. Since triathletes usually train pretty hard, physical activity levels can be quite low. Case in point: How many times have you done a long bike ride on Saturdays only to follow that up with an afternoon nap and then some more lounging around for the rest of the day? Well, if you want to lose weight and don't want to do it all by decreasing food intake, then you will have to increase your physical activity levels.

ENERGY EXPENDITURE FOR VARIOUS EXERCISES*

	59KG (130 LBS.) PERSON	70KG (155 LBS.) PERSON	82KG (180 LBS.) PERSON	93KG (205 LBS.) PERSON
Swimming laps (slow)	413	493	572	651
Swimming laps (fast)	590	704	817	931
Cycling (12–13.9 mph)	472	563	654	745
Cycling (14–15.9 mph)	590	704	817	931
Cycling (16–19 mph)	708	844	981	1,117
Cycling (>20 mph)	944	1,126	1,308	1,489
Running 6.0 mph (10 min / mile pace)	590	704	817	931
Running 6.7 mph (9 min / mile pace)	649	774	949	1,024
Running 7.5 mph (8 min / mile pace)	738	880	1,022	1,163
Running 8.6 mph (7 min / mile pace)	826	985	1,144	1,303
Running 10 mph (6 min / mile pace)	944	1,126	1,308	1,489
Running 10.9 mph (5.5 min / mile pace)	1,062	1,267	1,471	1,675
Weight lifting (light)	177	211	245	279

Source: NutriStrategy: Calories Burned During Exercise, nutristrategy.com/activitylist.htm.

* This table represents calories expended during one hour of activity.

Make Note: Healthy weight loss is 1 to 2 pounds per week (caloric deficit of 500 to 1,000 calories per day). For triathletes, the key is to lose weight at a rate that does not negatively affect performance. Too great of a caloric deficit, and you will not have the energy you need to train or race well.

Now, back to the issue of balancing weight loss with maintaining energy levels. If you want to lose weight, you should aim for 1 to 2 pounds per week. For athletes with just those last couple of pounds to lose, 1 pound per week is most appropriate. For athletes who have 15 to 20 (or more) pounds to lose, then 2 pounds per week is more appropriate. One to two pounds per week may not seem like much (especially in light of TV shows like *The Biggest Loser,* where contestants drop 10-plus pounds per week), but remember that you still want to maximize your training. If your goal is to lose weight to perform better/faster, but your training suffers because of low energy, then you probably will not achieve your goal even if you do lose weight. Let's do some math to determine your caloric deficit for the 1- to 2-pound-per-week weight-loss recommendation.

To lose 1 pound per week, your energy deficit will need to be 500 calories a day (500 calories x 7 days per week = 3,500 calories per week). To lose 2 pounds per week, your energy deficit needs to be 1,000 calories a day (1,000 calories x 7 days per week = 7,000 calories per week). A 1,000-calorie deficit can be difficult to achieve, and even more difficult to maintain. A caloric deficit greater than 1,000 calories a day will most certainly cause you to suffer from low energy levels, decreased training and performance, and a tendency to "fall off the weight-loss wagon" because you feel too hungry all the time.

When it comes to weight loss, patience is essential. The journey may seem long and slow, but if you do it the right way, you will achieve your weight-loss goals while maintaining optimal training and racing performance.

Achieving Weight Loss while Training

Here are some tips for what not to do, and how best to achieve your weight-loss goals while training.

First and foremost, there are times when it's acceptable to cut calories and there are other times when your body needs calories. Never skip breakfast—ever. Breakfast is "breaking the fast" from overnight. You use up most of your liver glycogen overnight, so you need to refuel your body in the morning. Your resting metabolism will also begin to slow down if you starve your body for a number of hours without food. Eight to ten hours is as long as you want to go without eating (and if you sleep less, then your fast should be for a shorter amount of time as well). Other times not to cut calories include during your pre-workout or pre-competition meal, during your training session or competition, and during your post-training or post-competition meal. Cutting calories during these times will only affect your performance and recovery.

The best time to cut calories is in the evening. This is also usually the most difficult time to cut calories, because people tend to snack at night. However, as an athlete, this is your best time to cut back a little. You should try to have consumed three-quarters of your daily calories by 4:00 p.m. If you eat most of your calories after that time, gradually change your eating habits to reach that goal. If you have a hard time cutting calories in the evening, you can also try making small decreases in your caloric intake throughout the day. Once again, though, don't cut those important calories that will affect your training and recovery.

Other Weight-Loss Tips

Here are some additional tips for losing weight:

- Use low-fat products (such as low-fat mayo or low-fat dairy products).

- Grill instead of fry.

- Eat more fiber (it increases satiety, or feelings of fullness).

- Cook at home more and eat out less.

- Look at nutrition info on food labels; you might be surprised at what (and how much) you actually eat.

- When eating out, look at the nutrition info for the restaurant's menu ahead of time and make healthy choices.

- Avoid appetizers.

- Allow yourself a cheat day or cheat meal on occasion (once a week at most).

- Eat everything in moderation (you can still have your favorite foods, such as pizza, but just not as much, or as often—or you need to put healthier ingredients on it).

- Eat more complex carbohydrates and fewer simple sugars.

- Eat only when you're hungry, not socially or out of boredom.

- Eat at a dining table and not in front of your TV.

- Plan your meals and menus ahead of time.

- Don't go grocery shopping when you are hungry. You are much more likely to buy unhealthier foods if you're starving while pushing your cart around the store.

- Don't go for long periods of time without eating (this will cause low blood sugar, which usually means you end up craving high-sugar, high-fat foods).

- Eat slowly because satiety (fullness) signals are delayed (it takes about 15 to 30 minutes for these signals to be integrated in the brain).

- Fill up on vegetables with meals.

- Avoid or minimize liquid calories (aside from those used as part of your nutrition training plan).

- Weigh yourself once a week, not daily, and always weigh yourself at the same time of day and with the same clothes on.

When I was a personal trainer, the first thing I had my clients do was keep a food diary. You might be surprised to learn what you actually eat. I always say that the best way to lose 5 pounds is to write down everything you eat (you may hesitate to grab that handful of cookies if you have to write down how many of them you ate—especially if you have to show that food diary to your triathlon coach). Be honest about this, though; otherwise, it defeats the whole purpose.

Metabolism and Body Fat Measurements

So many people complain about having a bad metabolism. As part of my job as a college professor, I do research in human metabolism and hunger and satiety signals. For the majority of people in the world, their metabolic rate is what you would expect to see given their age, gender, and weight, so stop using that as an excuse. Even if you do have a slightly slower metabolism than the average person, there's not much you can do to change that, so you will have to work with what God gave you.

If possible, get your body fat percentage measured. Too large of an energy deficit can lead to loss of skeletal muscle (protein will get pulled out of the muscle and made into new glucose to supply your brain and other organs with energy). Also, if you are just getting into triathlons and increasing your training, you may be gaining muscle mass. Therefore, the scale may actually show weight gain. Note that this gain could be more muscle, and you still may be losing fat.

If you get your body fat percentage measured, it should be with an accurate method. If you're going to do it, do it right. Spend the money it takes to get it done by Dual-Energy X-Ray Absorptiometry (DEXA), underwater weighing, or a BOD POD (similar principle to underwater weighing, but you don't have to get wet). If none of these is available to you, skinfold assessment can be okay, but only if it is performed by a trained technician. Bioelectrical Impedance Analysis (BIA) scales are instruments that you can stand on, or they are handheld units, popular at gyms. They can be used only to provide a rough estimate, as they are less accurate. The handheld BIA units are fairly cheap, but that's because they are the least accurate. If you get your body fat percentage measured, you should only check it one time per month after that to see if you are losing fat. More often than that and you're just likely to see the variation or error that exists with any method and not true changes in body fat.

A Note about Fad Diets

Most fad diets do not work or do not provide long-term results. The biggest mistake a triathlete can make is to go on a low-carbohydrate diet, which is perhaps one of the bigger fad diets out there today. Carbohydrates are simply too important; they fuel you for your workouts. You use your carbohydrate stores (glycogen) during exercise, and you need to replace those stores. If you are on a low-carb diet, you will not fully replace your glycogen stores after exercise, and, as a result, you will not have sufficient energy for your next workout.

Always try to remember that the ability to change your body weight boils down to that energy balance equation I mentioned previously. If you go on a low-carb, low-fat, or low-protein diet but maintain the same amount of calories, you will not lose weight; rather, it will likely affect your performance and/or recovery.

To recap:

1. Keep a food diary of what you are eating to help you avoid those unhealthy snacks that can really pack on the pounds.

2. Never skip breakfast.

3. Never cut back on food or fluids that are needed for successful training or competition.

4. Cut back on fat or sugar in your diet; don't cut back on nutrient-dense foods (i.e., fruits, vegetables, whole grains).

5. Stay away from fad diets.

6. Do not try to lose more than 1 to 2 pounds per week (caloric deficit of 500 to 1,000 calories per day).

7. Have patience; it can be a long and challenging journey.

CHAPTER 12

Supplements and Ergogenic Aids

Most people are familiar with dietary supplements. A supplement is any substance that is not a food or a drug but is designed to "supplement" the diet. It can be used to make up for a deficiency or to ensure adequate amounts of something. Supplements are not designed to replace food or be relied on to provide your body with everything that it needs.

An ergogenic aid is something that is designed to enhance athletic performance. This could be a dietary or nutritional supplement, although there are several different types of ergogenic aids. For example, ergogenic aids could include race wheels versus regular road wheels, or an aerodynamic helmet versus a regular riding helmet for touring. Since this book is about nutrition for triathletes, we will focus on dietary supplements as an ergogenic aid.

There are a few things you should know about supplements before we dive into some specific examples. First, I am not here to tell you whether or not to take a supplement, but I may give suggestions based on the scientific evidence (or lack thereof) for a particular product or type of supplement. Second, there are way too many supplements on the market to include all of them in this chapter. Therefore, I have chosen what I think are some of the more-common supplements to discuss here. Third, while supplements are commonly consumed among athletes, you should never take a supplement without doing a little research on the product first. Do not rely on testimonials—just because your super cyclist friend takes product "X" doesn't mean that it actually works, or that it will be good for you—or information from the manufacturer's website.

> **Make Note:** Do not rely on testimonials or manufacturer claims when determining the potential benefits of a supplement. Look to scientific research studies to see if the product has been proven effective.

Regulation and Safety of Supplements

One of the major issues with dietary supplements is that they are not regulated by the Food and Drug Administration (like the rest of our food supply), so FDA approval is not required before marketing a supplement. While this does not necessarily mean that all supplements are harmful, you should have your eyes wide open about possible problems with supplements if you currently take them, or plan on taking them in the future. The manufacturer is responsible for the safety of the product. Since supplements are not drugs, they do not have to undergo extensive research on safety and effectiveness, like drugs do. The manufacturer also does not have to prove the claims of their product (as long as they are not specific health claims). Therefore, the manufacturer can claim that their supplement increases muscle mass and strength without actually having to prove that their claim is true. Because of this, there are many, many products out there that simply do not work, or do not even come close to producing what they claim.

In addition to marketing and selling products that may not work, manufacturers also do not have to do quality-control testing. But just because they don't have to doesn't mean they all don't do it; some manufacturers (the more well-known and reputable ones) actually do test their products. Good Manufacturing Practices (GMP) are currently used for drug testing, and some supplement manufacturers also try to follow those. This basically means that the supplement met the established quality-control measures that currently exist.

In 2003, the United States Pharmacopeia (USP), a book that contains information about compound medicines and supplements, published guidelines on quality, purity, manufacturing practices, and ingredients of a given product or supplement. In order for manufacturers to be able to put the USP seal on their supplement, the following tests have to be passed:

1. The product is tested to verify that the ingredients and amounts of each ingredient that are listed on the label are correct.

2. The product is tested for contaminants.

3. The product is tested to ensure that the supplement will break down and release the ingredients once ingested in the body.

Therefore, if you are someone who uses supplements, you may want to look for the USP seal. If this seal is not present, it doesn't mean that the product isn't good; it just hasn't undergone that particular process of testing. Conversely, it's possible that a product without the USP seal is not good or safe for consumption.

General Categories of Supplements

There are a few major categories of ergogenic aids or supplements:

1. Prohormones and hormone releasers

2. Fat reducers

3. Anti-catabolics

4. Immune boosters

5. Micronutrients—vitamins and minerals

I have not included anabolics in this list because anabolic steroids are synthetic hormones and are not dietary supplements. Anabolics include things like testosterone and growth hormone, and are more common among strength athletes and bodybuilders than endurance athletes.

Prohormones and Hormone Releasers

Similarly, the first category—prohormones and hormone releasers—are not commonly used by endurance athletes because they are generally designed to increase strength and muscle mass. Prohormones are substances that are converted into an active hormone once ingested into the body. A very popular example of a prohormone is androstenedione ("andro"). The chemical structure of andro is only one conversion away from testosterone. The idea behind these prohormones—most of which are illegal—is that even though you aren't taking a synthetic hormone, you can still theoretically increase the amount of that hormone in your body by taking prohormones.

Hormone releasers are substances designed to stimulate the additional release of a specific hormone in the body. Some common examples include ornithine, arginine, and clonidine, which claim to increase growth-hormone levels in the body.

Fat Reducers

Fat reducers are designed to decrease appetite, increase metabolism (calorie burning), and/or block absorption of dietary fats. Common examples of fat reducers include caffeine, L-carnitine, ginseng, and ephedrine. Ephedrine is currently banned, so we will not cover it in this chapter. Most fat reducers are stimulants, which means they stimulate the central nervous system (CNS). In general, CNS stimulants will increase metabolic rate (so you burn more calories), stimulate or increase alertness and arousal, and have some effects on macronutrient metabolism. Stimulants also tend to decrease appetite. There are dangers associated with taking any type of stimulant, ranging from minor issues, such as feeling jittery and finding it difficult to concentrate, to more-serious side effects, like heart arrhythmias and other cardiovascular problems.

Caffeine is a CNS stimulant that has been studied in depth as an ergogenic aid. Many people think caffeine decreases appetite, but there is not a lot of research to support that. In studies on performance, however, caffeine has been shown to increase fat metabolism (which spares glycogen) and improve performance. It also increases the release of calcium in skeletal muscle, which leads to a more-efficient muscle contraction.

Unfortunately, caffeine can decrease blood flow to the heart, so people with heart conditions should exercise caution. One other problem with caffeine supplementation is that the doses needed to improve athletic performance are very high. Caffeine is a diuretic, so at high doses, it can cause dehydration. The high doses that are needed to increase performance can also cause you to feel shaky or jittery, which can negatively affect performance. Also, if you exercise for several hours, caffeine may cause you to push too hard early on, leaving you with nothing left in the tank at the end of your race. My recommendation for caffeine: If you consume it on a daily basis in moderate amounts, then you can continue to do so. It will not increase performance (unless you take really, really high doses of it), but it's probably not going to decrease performance in any way. In fact, if you are used to caffeine every day and decide to skip it on race day, you will likely have poorer performance because you will suffer from withdrawal symptoms.

L-carnitine (or carnitine) transports fats into a part of the cell where fat metabolism occurs. The claim for carnitine supplementation is that it will increase fat metabolism (and therefore spare muscle glycogen), which will increase performance and help with weight loss. Most of the research done on carnitine shows that it does not increase athletic performance and it does not help with weight loss. Your body can synthesize carnitine, so you already naturally produce the amount that your body needs. Providing your body with more carnitine does not seem to actually achieve the claims for the supplement.

Ginseng is an herbal remedy that is marketed as something that can increase fat metabolism. Some research supports improvements in VO^2 max (maximal aerobic capacity) after short-term supplementation (about six weeks), but most other studies do not show any effect on athletic performance. Some of the discrepancies in the research appear to be due to the varying degree of ginsenoside found in the ginseng root. Whether or not ginseng can lead to weight or fat loss also remains unknown.

Anti-Catabolics

Supplements that fall under the anti-catabolics category are also probably designed more for strength athletes interested in maintaining or increasing muscle mass, although some triathletes and other endurance athletes do supplement with these. Anti-catabolics are designed to prevent or decrease the breakdown of body tissues. This would decrease protein degradation and therefore potentially spare muscle mass. Some common anti-catabolics include some individual amino acid supplements (glutamine and leucine), as well as whey protein and the branched-chain amino acids (leucine, iso-leucine, and valine).

Since triathletes are endurance athletes, the supplements I will focus on here are those that are more commonly used by endurance athletes. From the categories above, this includes fat reducers, immune boosters, and micro-nutrients. This does not mean that triathletes do not take supplements that are anti-catabolics. Triathletes also take supplements that may not fit nicely into one of these three categories, or they may fit into more than one of these categories. We will finish the chapter with some common supplements that may not fall directly into one of these categories, so they will appear in the "other" category.

Immune Boosters

In chapter 13 I will discuss how a triathlete's immune system can be compromised during periods of heavy training, leaving them more prone to illness. Some common supplements designed and marketed to boost the immune system include colostrum, glutamine, and zinc.

Colostrum is actually the first milk that is produced after giving birth (produced by both humans and animals). It contains important antibodies and antimicrobial factors that are essential for newborns. In supplements, the most common kind is bovine colostrum. The claim of colostrum is that it boosts immune function and improves recovery from intense exercise. There have been only a few studies that have assessed the effectiveness of colostrum in athletes, and they tend to support better performance (able to exercise for longer) and decreased creatine kinase (CK) levels, which is a marker of muscle cell damage.

Glutamine is the most abundant amino acid in the body and there-fore has a number of important functions. Many systems in the body use glutamine, including the immune system, the small intestine, and kidney cells. Therefore, one of the marketing claims is that glutamine can bol-ster the immune system. Low levels of glutamine have also been detected during periods of overtraining, which would partially support this claim. Unfortunately, there is not a lot of research about how glutamine may affect the immune system. It has been shown to reduce infections post-marathon, but more research is needed to determine whether glutamine really does boost immune function. If you decide to take glutamine, it is usually recommended that you consume it after exercise, to prevent or decrease the chances of getting an infection.

Research does seem to support beneficial effects from taking zinc when you have a cold. Zinc lozenges reduce cold symptoms (sore throats, coughing, etc.), so if you get sick, you may want to reach for a zinc lozenge. There is little research on whether or not taking higher doses of zinc on a regular basis can boost the immune system and prevent illness. Prolonged exercise can decrease zinc levels, so it stands to reason that you may benefit from a little extra zinc. However, there is not enough research to support zinc supplementation at this time. If you are prone to illness, you may want to increase your zinc intake by eating some foods rich in zinc (oysters; sesame, pumpkin, and squash seeds; lean beef; lamb; wheat germ; and peanuts).

Micronutrients—Vitamins and Minerals

For this section, I will discuss the supplementation of individual vitamins or minerals. A daily multivitamin/mineral pill is considered a supplement. However, in this section, I will focus on supplementing with individual B vitamins or B vitamin complexes, chromium, and iron. I have already discussed some micronutrients in different sections in this chapter. However, some people take specific vitamins or minerals for reasons other than those described in chapters 4 and 5.

B vitamins and vitamin C supplements seem to be the most popular vitamin supplements among triathletes. While these vitamins are important for your body to function properly, you do not need to take megadoses of either. As I always tell athletes, unless you are deficient in a particular nutrient, taking supplements of that nutrient will not enhance your athletic performance. You will get B vitamins and vitamin C from various foods if you eat a relatively healthy diet, and you can also take a daily multivitamin pill as an insurance policy.

Make Note: As a general rule, unless you are deficient in a particular micronutrient, taking supplements of that micronutrient will not enhance your athletic performance.

Contrary to popular belief, taking extra B vitamins will not boost your energy levels or help you exercise better (unless for some uncommon reason you have developed a deficiency). The same goes for vitamin C. Taking supplements of vitamin C will not prevent you from getting a cold. Keep in mind that you cannot store extra B vitamins or vitamin C that you consume. Therefore, if you take in more than your body needs, you will simply excrete it in your urine. In fact, have you ever noticed that your urine is a bright yellow/greenish (almost neon yellow) color after you've taken a multivitamin or B vitamin complex? That color you see is the result of extra B2 (riboflavin) that is being excreted in your urine because your body didn't need it.

Chromium supplementation is not as popular among triathletes as it is with strength athletes. Chromium improves insulin sensitivity and is marketed as a product that can decrease body fat, increase muscle mass, and increase metabolism. Most studies have shown no effect on body weight and lean mass, though. Those few that have shown results have experienced very small or minimal amounts of weight loss.

Iron is a popular supplement simply because so many people have an iron deficiency (female athletes in particular). However, it can be toxic at high doses, and your body is very efficient at storing iron, so I wouldn't recommend taking supplements unless your physician has diagnosed you with anemia and has specifically suggested iron supplements. If you are not deficient in iron, taking supplements will not further increase RBC (red blood cell) production or oxygen-carrying capacity in your body, so it will not improve your performance. However, if you suffer from anemia due to low iron, then supplementation will improve your athletic performance and bring it back up to where it should have been.

Other Supplements

Coenzyme Q10 (CoQ10), also known as ubiquinone, helps with energy production in the body and has some antioxidant function as well. The claim for CoQ10 supplementation is that it will enhance endurance-exercise performance and decrease free-radical damage. Most research studies show that CoQ10 does not improve athletic performance. There may be some antioxidant benefits with supplementation, but the only research to support this is in animal models and not in humans.

Much like CoQ10, pyruvate is marketed as a supplement that can increase energy production in the body. Very high doses of pyruvate have been shown to increase time to exhaustion during exercise, but this only works for exercise lasting one to two hours. Moderate doses of pyruvate do not have any affect on performance. Therefore, with realistic doses of pyruvate, you more than likely will not get any performance-enhancing effects from supplementation.

Glycerol is actually part of the structure of a triglyceride, but it is marketed as a "hyperhydrating" agent for athletes. Glycerol supplementation does increase ADH (anti-diuretic hormone) levels, which then leads to fluid retention. The research on glycerol supplementation does show improved endurance time, a lower heart rate, and a lower core body temperature. However, this only works in well-trained athletes and in hot, humid climates. It also may only help if substantial dehydration is occurring. Finally, since glycerol increases ADH levels, athletes are at a greater risk for hyponatremia (discussed in chapter 6), which can be deadly.

Multiple studies claim that branched-chain amino acids (BCAAs)— leucine, isoleucine, and valine—actually improve endurance performance. BCAAs are metabolized differently in the body than other amino acids, and are therefore used preferentially as a protein energy source in skeletal muscle. Additionally, BCAAs purportedly delay central fatigue and maintain mental performance. Some studies have shown that BCAA supplementation improved marathon performance (but only for those triathletes needing more than three hours to finish); another study showed that BCAAs helped to decrease glycogen breakdown during and after exercise. A two-week supplementation study also showed improvements in a time trial in trained cyclists.

However, there are also a number of studies that show no improvements with either acute or chronic BCAA supplementation, so the choice is up to you. There do not seem to be any negative side effects with BCAA supplementation, so if you are looking to try something, this may be a good place to start. You can also get BCAAs from several food sources (red meat, poultry, eggs, dairy products, and most other meats), so if you do not want to spend money on supplements, you can relax, knowing that you are getting BCAAs from a healthy, balanced diet.

The Importance of Researching Your Supplements

I haven't even come close to covering all of the supplementation products that are available today for triathletes. If there is a supplement that you are considering taking, do your homework first. Reading product advertisements or the information found on manufacturer websites is not doing your homework. Remember that manufacturers do not have to prove the claims they make about athletic performance. Therefore, you need to do a little research on your own before you decide whether or not purchasing a supplement will be beneficial for you.

I recommend that you do a search for research studies (that are published in respectable journals) on PubMed (pubmed.org) and/or Google Scholar (scholar.google.com). Read several articles (if they are available) and then form your own opinion. Oftentimes you will see some studies showing benefits and other studies that don't. If that is the case and you are really uncertain, I recommend you seek out a nutrition specialist (such as a registered dietitian) who has experience in research and can critique the articles to give you a solid recommendation.

CHAPTER 13

Illness and Injury

included this chapter because I am one of those unfortunate individuals who has a tendency to get sick quite often, especially during heavy periods of training. The absolute worst is getting sick right before a big race. While illness during training is something you can work around, illness right before a race leaves you with few options.

It was always a dream of mine to run the Boston Marathon. I qualified for it and trained hard so I would have a good race. Mostly, though, I just wanted to soak up the positive experience of doing this historic race. Sadly, I came down with a monster of a cold two days before the race. I walked downtown to pick up my race packet the day before the marathon and was so exhausted by the time I made it back to my hotel, I didn't think there was any way I could race. Of course, my frugal side came out and I decided I had to race because I had traveled all the way there, spent all the money for the trip, and had trained hard for four months. I ran with Kleenex in both hands and stuffed into my shirt pocket, and somehow managed to get through the race. The entire day was brutal, though, and I decided that this would be the last time I'd race when I was really sick (unless I happen to qualify for Kona, and then I'd race in any condition!).

If, like me, you are prone to illness, the unfortunate news is that some of this is pure genetics. If you do everything "right" to try to protect yourself against illness and you still get sick frequently, you can thank your parents for that one. Regardless of the cards you have been dealt, however, there are still things you can do to prevent or lower your risk of getting sick.

Now I don't want you to think that exercise is the enemy here. Studies have shown that exercise can actually improve immune function—up to a certain point. The problems occur when athletes start doing really heavy training. Heavy exercise (very high volumes and/or very high intensities) tends to suppress immune function. This occurs in two different ways: acutely and chronically. Let's start with the acute effect. A single bout of very hard exercise can transiently suppress the immune system, allowing infectious diseases (usually viral illnesses) to attack. This is why so many athletes get sick after ultra marathons and half or full Ironman triathlons. The chronic effect occurs with sustained heavy training or overtraining that gradually weakens an athlete's immune system. This leads to more frequent illness and injury.

Overtraining

So why are triathletes more prone to getting sick than the average couch potato? Well, think of exercise as a form of stress for the body. Small to moderate amounts of this are actually beneficial, but too much will negatively affect different systems in your body, including your immune system. Because of the nature of our sport, triathletes run the risk of overtraining. What does this mean, exactly? Overtraining occurs when exercise exceeds the body's ability to recover. There are signs and symptoms of overtraining, including muscle fatigue, persistent muscle soreness, changes in mood (tension, depression, anger, fatigue, irritability), depleted muscle glycogen stores, increased resting heart rate, increased cortisol levels, decreased appetite, sleep disturbances, head colds, immunosuppression, increased incidence of injuries, and decreased performance.

If you feel some of these symptoms, you may be overtrained. The goal for every triathlete should be to prevent overtraining from occurring. This is difficult for some triathletes, especially the competitive ones who push themselves to their limit. There's a fine line between maximum training for benefit and overtraining. Usually it just takes experience and practice to know where that line is. If you are overtrained, you need to rest until you recover. Of course, no triathlete likes to hear that, but there's not much else that you can do. It can take several weeks (or months) to recover from overtraining.

The longer you have overtrained, the more rest time you need. If you have overtrained for a few weeks, then three to seven days of rest is usually sufficient (followed by a lower volume of training). If you have overtrained for longer (say, a few months), then it may take several weeks or months of rest and reduced training to fully recover.

> **Make Note:** A triathlete's immune system can be compromised or weakened during periods of heavy training. Maintaining a healthy diet every day and getting plenty of sleep is important to ward off illnesses.

Your immune system provides a defense against bacteria, parasites, viruses, and tumor cells. Unfortunately, if you do a high volume and intensity of training, you may have a compromised immune system. Because of this, you may get sick more frequently; in addition, the symptoms, severity, and length of illness can also be increased exponentially when you train heavily. What might be just a minor cold that slows you down a little during other times of the year can become a major cold that really knocks you on your butt during heavy periods of training.

The question then becomes: Do I take time off to hopefully get healthy faster (but risk losing fitness), or do I push through this and continue training so I don't lose fitness (even though I'll risk being sick for much longer)? The answer is . . . actually, I don't have the answer for you. (Sorry—such buildup for a nonanswer.) It really depends on the individual and how sick they are.

If the illness seems pretty minor and you feel like you have the energy, do a light workout and see how you recover afterward. Sometimes you will feel pretty good during the training session, but then afterward you'll feel totally whipped and realize (after it's too late) that you've trained too hard. So start with a light training session and see how you recover from it before planning your next workout.

In other instances, your illness may be severe enough that just getting out of bed seems like a struggle. If that is the case, do not exercise at all. You may find that you have a little energy—enough to get a workout in—but it will wipe you out and slow down your recovery process. The end result is that you will have done some subpar training (that probably didn't give you any benefits anyway), and you will end up being sicker for a longer period of time.

Boosting Your Immune System

Even if you are not overtraining, your immune system can be compromised because of the high volume and intensity of exercise that you, as a triathlete, do. Here are a few nutrition hints for bolstering your immune system, especially during the times of year when you do heavy training and/or run the risk of overtraining:

1. Get adequate calories. When you're in the midst of heavy training, it's not the time to cut calories or try to lose weight. First of all, triathletes usually cut too many calories, which means their training really suffers. If you aren't getting enough calories, your immune system can become weaker, ultimately leaving you more prone to illness.

2. Eat immediately after training. You should do this as part of your recovery from exercise anyway, but it also helps your immune system. A study done on military recruits—where investigators either gave no calories, carbohydrates alone, or a combination of carbohydrates and protein after exercise—showed that the group of recruits consuming the combination of carbohydrates and protein right after exercise had fewer medical visits due to bacterial and viral infections, fewer muscle and joint problems, and less heat exhaustion. While this is just one study, it does reinforce what I've said in previous chapters about eating properly immediately after training.

3. Get enough essential amino acids. A final nutritional concern for bolstering the immune system is to make sure you get enough essential amino acids, necessary to repair muscle and tissue damage from training, and for making proteins for the immune system. Therefore, it's vital that you eat quality protein sources (complete proteins) to make sure you're providing the right types and quantities of amino acids for your body.

Nutrition and Your Immune System

When it comes to your immune system, the best advice I can give is to try not to be a hero. You will not lose fitness, get totally out of shape, or gain a bunch of weight if you take a few days off. Sometimes this can be a difficult concept to pound into a triathlete's head, because most endurance athletes are so accustomed to pushing hard and doing high volumes of training. You really will bounce back quickly if you take care of yourself when you are sick and get plenty of rest.

There are some additional nutrition tips I can give you to help with the recovery process. First, make sure you get enough fluids. Most people don't really feel like eating or drinking when they are sick, but you need to force yourself to get enough fluids. Make sure you get at least 8 to 10 cups a day of fluid if you aren't training, and even more than that if you are. Try to eat some fruits and vegetables so you get a variety of micronutrients, and also try to meet your daily needs for protein (necessary to fight off whatever virus or bacteria that plagues you).

Despite what many people think, vitamin C does not seem to help you recover more quickly from a cold; in fact, many studies show no benefit whatsoever. Therefore, you actually don't need to take a whole bunch of vitamin C when you get sick. On the other hand, research does seem to support beneficial effects from taking zinc when you have a cold. Zinc lozenges reduce cold symptoms (sore throats, coughing, etc.), so if you get sick, you may want to reach for a zinc lozenge. Unfortunately, chronic zinc supplementation does not appear to help with prevention of illness unless you are not getting enough zinc in your diet.

There are several micronutrients that play a role in the immune system, so make sure you get the recommended amounts of them (for food sources for these nutrients, please see chapters 4 and 5). These micronutrients include vitamin C, vitamin A, vitamin B6, iron, zinc, and selenium. In short, eat a variety of healthy foods (fruits, vegetables, whole grains, legumes, nuts and seeds, and lean meats) and take a daily multivitamin/mineral pill to ensure that you cover all of these nutrient needs.

In addition to eating a healthy diet and getting plenty of rest, there are a number of supplements that are designed and marketed specifically to boost the immune system. We have already covered these in detail in chapter 12.

Some final tips to try to prevent or minimize your susceptibility to illness include:

1. Wash your hands frequently to prevent the spread of germs and infections.

2. Get plenty of sleep in the weeks leading up to your race and during your heaviest training periods.

3. Try to avoid circumstances where you will be in contact with huge crowds and groups of people (where you can pick up germs easily) in the weeks leading up to your race.

4. Traveling seems to be a breeding ground for illness. Try to avoid travel (unless it's just you in your car or on your bike) in the weeks leading up to your race.

5. Make sure you eat plenty of fruits and vegetables and take your daily multivitamin/mineral pill so you will get an adequate amount of antioxidants.

6. Do not restrict calories in the weeks leading up to your race, as this can compromise your immune system.

Injuries

This section of the chapter deals with injuries often experienced by triathletes.

Once during an Ironman event, I noticed that a fellow competitor had just finished pumping up his bike (with his own pump) in the bike transition area. After pumping, he started off at a light jog to take his pump back to his vehicle. He went about three steps before letting out a cry and coming up hobbling. He had pulled a hamstring on race morning—just hours before the gun was set to go off. I actually heard the pop/ripping sound of his muscle and knew that his day was over before it had even begun. I still feel bad for this man every time I think about what happened to him. Hopefully any injury you experience will occur during training and not on race morning, but either way, injuries will happen, so you need to be prepared.

Since this book is geared toward nutrition for triathletes, we will not spend time on the physiology of injuries and how to recover from them. For most triathletes, injury is just part of the sport. Specifically, overuse injuries are quite common because of the repetitive nature of each of the disciplines within the sport of triathlon. Some common injuries include:

- Running: Tendonitis, plantar fasciitis, iliotibial band syndrome (ITBS), patellofemoral pain syndrome (aka, "runner's knee"), shin splints, stress fractures, Achilles tendonitis, and muscle pulls (hamstring in particular).

- Cycling: Hand and/or foot numbness, knee pain, ITBS, and piriformis syndrome (piriformis muscle compresses or irritates the sciatic nerve).

- Swimming: Biceps tendonitis, "swimmer's shoulder" (tendonitis to the rotator cuff), and other shoulder injuries (such as rotator cuff impingement).

Because triathletes train in three different disciplines, their risk for developing an injury is greater than for many other athletes.

Nutrition for Injuries

Before I get to some nutrition tips for injuries, I want to give just one piece of non-nutrition advice for treating injuries: rest. Triathletes always push the envelope with training, but if you do not allow your body adequate time to heal from injuries, it will take much longer for you to feel 100 percent again. Here are some things you can eat that may help prevent injuries from occurring or help you to recover more quickly from an injury.

Stress fractures are common among runners, especially females. If you are prone to stress fractures, you should try to get more calcium, phosphorus, and vitamin D in your diet. These are some of the micronutrients that are important for bone function. Low-fat and fat-free dairy products are an excellent way to get more of these important nutrients. For some of the other common injuries that involve joints, tendons, and ligaments, make sure you

26

get enough omega-3 fatty acids (cold-water fatty fish, fish oil, flax seeds, flax oil, and walnuts), vitamin C, and copper, because they have an important role in collagen formation and wound healing. Collagen synthesis or formation is important because it is used to make connective tissue for tendons, ligaments, cartilage, bones, and teeth.

There are some other micronutrients that play a role in wound healing and new tissue development, including zinc, sulfur, vitamin B12, vitamin B9 (folate), and vitamin B7 (biotin). Eat a variety of healthy foods and take your daily multivitamin/mineral pill to ensure that you provide your body with all of the micronutrients it needs to prevent or recover from injury.

Make Note: If you are prone to stress fractures, try getting more calcium, phosphorus, and vitamin D in your diet.

These micronutrients are all important for injury prevention and, to some extent, for recovery from injury. In addition to these, if you are already injured, make sure you get a little extra protein in your diet. The amino acids from dietary protein can be used to synthesize new body proteins (build new tissue) in order to repair and replace the old and damaged tissue (muscle, tendons, or ligaments).

Finally, if you do have to take some time off or cut back on your training in order to heal from your injury, make sure you adjust your caloric intake accordingly. You will need some extra calories to recover from your injury, but you will probably need fewer calories overall, because your volume of training has decreased. Triathletes do not like taking time off, so if weight gain occurs during that rest time, it's even more stressful for the athlete. Just try to eat healthy and cut back on your caloric intake a little to make up for the extra couch time.

CHAPTER 14

Frequently Asked Questions (FAQs)

Once triathletes learn that I am a sports nutritionist, I usually get bombarded with questions. They range from questions about everyday nutrition for optimal health to very specific nutrition issues triathletes may face during training or racing. Here I have documented some of the more-common questions that I get, along with my answers. Chances are, you may have at least a couple of these same questions. Hopefully this chapter will provide some additional clarification for you.

Travel

Q: *I travel for most of my races and find myself completely changing my nutrition while on the road. What do you suggest to help me stick to my nutrition plan and also to reduce my chances of getting sick?*

A: For most triathletes, travel is just a part of racing. This is especially true for half and full Ironman races. Traveling to a race venue can be great—new scenery, new people, new surroundings. On the other hand, travel can also complicate things, such as your nutrition plan. If you are like most people, your eating patterns will change when you travel. Most people do not follow quite as healthy a diet when they travel, particularly as dining out is almost a necessity.

Unfortunately, this usually means meals that are higher in calories, fat, and sodium than what you are used to. It may also mean not eating at your normal times, not consuming your usual water intake, and consuming more alcohol or junk food than usual. The longer you are away from home, the harder it is to try to stick to your typical eating patterns. The key to maintaining a healthy diet on the road is planning. You can access almost every restaurant on the Internet these days, and most of them have nutrition information. You can use this information to plan your eating destinations during your trip. This may seem silly to many of you, but you will eat healthier if you have a game plan for your travel days.

Planning ahead also allows you to bring along nonperishable items on your trip. Your last trip to the grocery store should include the purchase of those foods you plan to bring with you. This will help you plan out healthy snacks (and save you some money in the process). There's nothing wrong with packing some fruits and vegetables, protein bars, mixed nuts, etc., in your carry-on. You can also check ahead to find out if you will have access to a fridge or microwave at your hotel. Again, this information can help you plan what foods or beverages to bring with you, or what to buy at the local grocery store upon arrival at your destination.

As much as possible, try to eat at the same times of day you usually do, and stick to the meal sizes that you are used to. For example, if you don't usually eat 1,000 calories for lunch, don't do it when you travel. If you don't usually eat 500 calories' worth of ice cream in the afternoon, don't do it when you travel. Instead, eat meals that contain a similar calorie content to what you are used to, and eat snacks (such as protein bars) that you would normally eat at home. Also, drink water at the same frequency you do at home. If you're used to carrying around a bottle of water with you, then do the same when you're on the road.

As for the second part of this question, travel seems to increase a triathlete's chances of getting sick. You are simply being exposed to more people and places, which means more viruses and bacteria. Make sure you get adequate amounts of vitamins and minerals, and if you are prone to illness or feel something coming on, then I suggest taking a zinc lozenge or two. Also make sure you wash your hands frequently and get plenty of sleep.

Tapering

Q: *I never know what I should eat during a taper. Should my nutrition and caloric intake change during a two- to three-week taper?*

A: First of all, let's define this term. A taper is a reduction in exercise (either volume, intensity, or both) for a period of time before a race. For longer-distance races (half and full Ironman), a taper is probably part of your training plan. If it's not, then it should be. Strange things can happen when someone tapers for a race. In general, the triathlete feels terrible during the first few days or week of the taper. This is followed by a few days to a week where the athlete finally feels like they are recovering from their hard training. This should bring you close to your race, so the last few days of your taper leave you feeling ready and rejuvenated for race day.

When triathletes think about tapering, they are usually concerned with how much to decrease training volume and intensity, and how long they should taper for. Do not overlook nutrition during this period. During the first week of a taper, appetite usually goes up despite the fact that your volume of training has gone down. This seems counterintuitive, but it is your body trying to tell you something. Part of recovery is to completely refuel the body and maximize carbohydrate stores and complete muscle recovery (protein synthesis for new muscle and for repairing muscle). So, if you feel hungrier, then your body probably needs the nutrients.

On the flip side, high training volumes can suppress appetite. So, when you first start tapering, your appetite might go up simply because you are not as fatigued from training. It's important not to overeat during this period because you do not want to gain weight in the two to three weeks before your race. Try to listen to your body and distinguish between hunger and appetite. Hunger is the physiological feeling that you get when you are genuinely hungry. Appetite is the desire to eat—not the need to eat. You should eat when you're hungry, but it's best to try not to eat when you simply "want" to eat (but your body doesn't really need anything).

Appetite usually rears its ugly head in the evenings, so be careful of "TV eating" (eating huge amounts of food without even realizing it because you're concentrating on the boob tube). You also want to be sure to eat plenty of carbohydrates and protein during your taper so your body can recover and restore as well. If you decide to cut back on calories because your training volume has decreased, then cut back on fat calories first.

During the second and third week of a taper (if you're doing a three-week taper), your appetite may go down a little, but you still have to be careful not to overeat. It's easy to do because you may be used to eating huge amounts of food, but with a large drop in training, you do need to cut back on your caloric intake.

However, make sure you do eat when you are hungry. The absolute worst thing you can do is under-eat because you're afraid of gaining weight. Not eating enough will mean that you haven't fueled your body for race day, and it will affect your performance. One to three weeks before your race is not the time to try to lose weight. If you do see weight loss in the last couple of weeks, make sure you drink plenty of fluids and increase your carbohydrate and protein intake slightly.

The take-home message here is to listen to your body; it will tell you when you need food. It's important for you to try to recognize the difference between the need to eat and the desire to eat. One easy way to do this is by thinking of vegetables. If you're sitting on the couch in the evening and you want to eat (and are trying to decide if it's actual hunger and not merely appetite), allow yourself to eat all the fresh vegetables you want. If you're hungry, then you'll eat them. If you would rather not eat than have to eat some broccoli and carrot sticks, then you probably aren't actually hungry.

Late-Night Eating

Q: *I can't seem to stop snacking in the evening, even though I know it's not healthy for me. What can I do to prevent late-night cravings?*

A: One of the no-no's for people trying to lose weight (or maintain weight) is late-night snacking; however, it's a bit different for triathletes who train several hours each day. During intense periods of training I often wake up during the night, extremely hungry, and I can't seem to fall back asleep until I put something in my belly. If you are legitimately hungry, then you should eat something in the evenings. However, if you reach for junk food (chips, desserts), then you're not doing yourself any favors.

The key is to determine whether or not you actually need some additional calories. If you know you are going to eat something in the evening, then make sure you don't overeat at dinner so you've "saved" some calories for your snack. Here are some tips to make sure that you don't overeat late in the evening, and that you eat healthy snacks:

1. Do not eat while sitting in front of the TV or computer. If you want a snack, prepare it in your kitchen and sit at your dining room table to eat. If you eat in front of a TV or computer, you will have a tendency to overeat because you're not really paying attention to how much you're chowing down.

2. Drink plenty of water. Sometimes when you are thirsty, you can mistake that for hunger. Drink a glass or two of water in the evening. If you still feel hungry after that, then go and make yourself a healthy snack.

3. Avoid high-sugar, high-salt, or high-fat foods. When you have a desire to eat (but are not actually hungry), you usually crave sugar, salt, and fat. If you would rather skip the snack if your options are a piece of whole-wheat toast or some fruit and string cheese, then you probably don't actually need any additional calories.

4. Eat nutrient-dense foods rather than energy-dense foods. This is an extension of point three. Here are some examples of good snacks for the evening, starting with my favorite:

   - Cottage cheese (low-fat or fat-free) plus fresh fruit (you choose—mango, any type of berry, pineapple, peaches, plums, and melons—they all taste great).
   - Cereal and milk (make sure it's not a high-sugar cereal).
   - Protein bar or shake.
   - Smoothie (made with yogurt, fruit, milk, water, and/or protein powder—the protein powder will help make you feel full).
   - Any fresh vegetables (if you need some dip or dressing, try fat-free Ranch).
   - Some walnuts or almonds with any type of fresh fruit.
   - Whole-wheat toast or bagel with natural peanut butter.
   - Glass of low-fat or fat-free milk (or low-fat chocolate milk, if you want to treat yourself occasionally).
   - String cheese or yogurt.

The take-home message here is that if you feel hungry in the evening, you should eat. Just make sure you're actually hungry (and not eating out of boredom), and try to eat healthy, balanced snacks. If you go to bed feeling really full, then you probably overate.

Pre-Race Jitters

Q: *I am so nervous on race morning that nothing sounds appealing. What can I eat when I feel this way, or what can I do to calm my stomach?*

A: One of the hardest things to do when you are nervous is eat something. If you are like most triathletes, you get nervous before a race, especially if it is your first race or a big race that you've been training hard for. When a person gets nervous, his appetite usually disappears. In fact, it is common for a nervous athlete to feel nauseous even at the mere thought of eating something. This can make it pretty difficult to consume your pre-race meal. This is when you need to have a Plan B. That bagel or cereal might have sounded good when you were coming up with your nutrition plan, but if you can't choke it down on race day, you need to have another option.

For many triathletes, liquids are the answer. In general, liquid calories are easier to get down (and keep down) when you are nervous. Boost and Ensure both have a decent amount of calories and carbohydrates, so either one would be a good alternative. You should try this during a couple of training days to make sure you can tolerate it.

Another thing you can try on race morning is taking a short walk. For some reason movement seems to calm a person down a little. This may help just enough for you to be able to get some calories in your stomach before the gun goes off.

Stomach Savers during Racing

Q: *During my full Ironman races, I always get nauseous and lose my appetite. What are some things I can do to prevent or fix those problems during my race?*

A: During long-distance races (full Ironman and sometimes half Ironman), athletes will often experience some GI distress. Minimally, this can include nausea or a lack of appetite. On a bad day, this can mean diarrhea and/or vomiting. We've all seen these athletes (or we've actually been that athlete), and we wonder what went wrong. We could assume that they made some nutrition-related mistake, but that's not always the case. Sometimes what works during training simply doesn't sit well on race day.

I know a number of individuals who can tolerate solid foods just fine during training but can only take in liquids and gels on race day. Unfortunately, it usually takes experiencing this in a race to find out if you're that kind of person. Flavor fatigue is also quite common during a full Ironman race, and can lead to nausea and a loss of appetite. (See chapter 10 for suggestions on how to avoid or deal with flavor fatigue on race day.)

There are probably some other explanations for nausea and loss of appetite during a long race, but, regardless of the reason, you need to be able to deal with it. Not eating is simply not an option (at least, if you want to finish). Here are a few tricks of the trade that may work for you:

1. Pepto-Bismol chewable tablets are pink magic: They have saved me on a number of occasions. If you have an upset stomach, chew a tablet or two, and it may completely calm your stomach down.

2. Salty food: This can include any number of foods, as long as they are not also sweet. For some reason, eating something really salty seems to help with flavor fatigue and may actually restore your appetite. If you feel sick during the bike portion of a half or full Ironman race, I recommend eating beef jerky or crackers (Combos also work pretty well). If it is during the run portion of your race, then stick to the chicken broth that is provided (for full Ironman races), or pretzels.

3. Flat cola: This is served on every Ironman course and considered "liquid gold" by some. I personally do not care for it, but I know many triathletes who claim this has saved their race. It provides carbs, and for many, can calm an upset stomach and help with flavor fatigue.

4. Skipping the sports drinks: A friend of mine recently finished a half Ironman and she said it was the first race where she hadn't experienced some type of GI distress. The only thing she did differently for this race was to skip the sports drinks. She made sure she took in enough carbohydrates and fluids, and also took

salt tablets to get electrolytes. It is possible that sports drinks and sweet-tasting foods can lead to quicker flavor fatigue, which may lead to nausea or other GI complications. Therefore, if you have some GI distress, try cutting back on the sports drinks. Just make sure you "make up" for those calories, carbohydrates, fluids, and electrolytes with other food/drink items.

Nausea with Daily Multivitamin/Mineral Pill

Q: *When I take my daily multivitamin/mineral pill, I get nauseous. Is this common, and what can I do to avoid it?*
A: This is actually quite common. It generally happens when people take their pill on an empty stomach, or with their first meal of the day. For some reason, taking it on an empty stomach can cause temporary nausea. The fix for this is simple: Make sure you take your multivitamin/mineral pill with food. If you try taking it with breakfast and still feel a little sick, then wait until lunch to take your pill.

CHAPTER 15

Top Ten Nutrition Tips for Triathletes

I have made several important points throughout this book and have provided a great deal of nutrition information. Here is a Top Ten list of what I feel are the most important take-home messages:

1. **Carbohydrate intake during training or racing should be 60 to 70 grams per hour.**
   - No carbohydrates are necessary for sixty minutes or less of exercise.
   - Up to 90 grams per hour is optimal for any athlete who can handle that amount and is training/racing for three to four hours or more.

2. **Perform sweat trials to determine fluid needs during training.**
   - Do these trials for all three disciplines of triathlon, and try to match intake with losses.
   - Perform trials in climate conditions similar to what is expected on race day.

3. **Consume 1 cup of fluid every ten to twenty minutes during training or racing.**
   - Most triathletes can handle about 4 cups of fluid per hour on the bike, and about 2 to 3 cups of fluid per hour on the run.

4. **Electrolyte or salt tablets should be taken if exercising for longer than four hours, and/or if exercising for at least three hours in a hot, humid environment.**
   - Sodium content in these tablets varies greatly, so make sure you read the label carefully. Most triathletes should not go over 1,000 milligrams of sodium per hour.

5. **For proper recovery, remember 1.2 grams of carbohydrate per kilogram of body weight, and 6 to 20 grams of essential amino acids immediately after training or racing.**
   - This recovery meal should be consumed within fifteen to thirty minutes after exercise.
   - This recovery meal should also be consumed every hour for the first three to four hours, or you should consume a larger meal two hours post-exercise.

6. **Keep fiber and fat intake low or avoid altogether before, during, and right after training or racing.**
   - Fiber and fat can cause GI distress and will slow down the digestion and absorption of other nutrients.

7. **Pre-race or pre-training meal should be rich in carbohydrates.**
   - Recommended carbohydrate intake is 1.5 to 4.0 grams per kilogram of body weight, about two to four hours before exercise.

8. **Never skip breakfast or train after an overnight fast.**
   - Your liver is depleted of glycogen after an overnight fast, so you need to eat in order to have carbohydrates available for exercise.

9. **Never try anything new on race day.**
   - Always practice your race-day nutrition during several training sessions to make sure your body responds well to your nutrition plan.

10. **Follow a healthy, balanced diet to get all of the nutrients you need on a daily basis.**

- Consume about 50 to 65 percent of calories from carbohydrates (or 6 to 10 grams per kilogram of body weight).
- Consume about 15 to 20 percent of calories from protein (or 1.2 to 2.0 grams per kilogram of body weight).
- Consume about 20 to 35 percent of calories from fat.
- Eat a variety of fruits and vegetables, low-fat or fat-free dairy products, whole grains, and lean protein sources to ensure that you get all of the vitamins and minerals that your body needs.
- Total water consumption is about 3.7 liters per day for men and 2.7 liters per day for women.

Appendix

Common Abbreviations

AA = amino acid

AI = adequate intake

AMDR = acceptable macronutrient distribution range

BCAA = branched-chain amino acid

DRI = dietary reference intake

DV = daily value

EAA = essential amino acid

GI = gastrointestinal (this is your digestive system or digestive tract)

HR = heart rate

IM = Ironman triathlon

MCT = medium-chain triglyceride

MUFA = monounsaturated fatty acid

PUFA = polyunsaturated fatty acid

RDA = recommended dietary allowance

SFA = saturated fatty acid

SUMMARY OF DIETARY REFERENCE INTAKES FOR VITAMINS

	VITAMIN A (μg/d)	VITAMIN C (mg/d)	VITAMIN D (μg/d)	VITAMIN E (mg/d)	B1 (THIAMINE) (mg/d)	B2 (RIBOFLAVIN) (mg/d)	B3 (NIACIN) (mg/d)
MALES							
19–30 years old	**900**	**90**	**15**	**15**	**1.2**	**1.3**	**16**
31–50 years old	**900**	**90**	**15**	**15**	**1.2**	**1.3**	**16**
51–70 years old	**900**	**90**	**15**	**15**	**1.2**	**1.3**	**16**
FEMALES							
19–30 years old	**700**	**75**	**15**	**15**	**1.1**	**1.1**	**14**
31–50 years old	**700**	**75**	**15**	**15**	**1.1**	**1.1**	**14**
51–70 years old	**700**	**75**	**15**	**15**	**1.1**	**1.1**	**14**

Recommended Dietary Allowances (RDAs) in **bold type** and Adequate Intakes (AIs) in ordinary type followed by an asterisk (*).

Information for this table obtained from the DRI reports (www.nap.edu) from the Institute of Medicine of the National Academies.

SUMMARY OF DIETARY REFERENCE INTAKES FOR MINERALS

	CALCIUM (mg/d)	CHROMIUM (μg/d)	COPPER (μg/d)	FLUORIDE (mg/d)	IODINE (μg/d)	IRON (mg/d)	MAGNESIUM (mg/d)
MALES							
19–30 years old	**1,000**	35*	**900**	4*	150	**8**	**400**
31–50 years old	**1,000**	35*	**900**	4*	150	**8**	**420**
51–70 years old	**1,000**	30*	**900**	4*	150	**8**	**420**
FEMALES							
19–30 years old	**1,000**	25*	**900**	3*	150	**18**	**310**
31–50 years old	**1,000**	25*	**900**	3*	150	**18**	**320**
51–70 years old	**1,200**	20*	**900**	3*	150	**8**	**320**

Recommended Dietary Allowances (RDAs) in **bold type** and Adequate Intakes (AIs) in ordinary type followed by an asterisk (*).

Information for this table obtained from the DRI reports (www.nap.edu) from the Institute of Medicine of the National Academies.

(PYRIDOXAL) (mg/d)	B9 (FOLATE) (μg/d)	B12 (COBALAMIN) (μg/d)	B5 (PANTOTHENIC ACID) (mg/d)	B7 (BIOTIN) (μg/d)	CHOLINE (mg/d)
1.3	400	2.4	5*	30*	550*
1.3	400	2.4	5*	30*	550*
1.7	400	2.4	5*	30*	550*
1.3	400	2.4	5*	30*	425*
1.3	400	2.4	5*	30*	425*
1.3	400	2.4	5*	30*	425*

μg/d = micrograms per day
mg/d = milligrams per day

MANGANESE (mg/d)	MOLYBDENUM (μg/d)	PHOSPHORUS (mg/d)	SELENIUM (μg/d)	ZINC (mg/d)	POTASSIUM (g/d)	SODIUM (g/d)	CHLORIDE (g/d)
2.3*	45	700	55	11	4.7*	1.5*	2.3*
2.3*	45	700	55	11	4.7*	1.5*	2.3*
2.3*	45	700	55	11	4.7*	1.5*	2.3*
1.8*	45	700	55	8	4.7*	1.5*	2.3*
1.8*	45	700	55	8	4.7*	1.5*	2.3*
1.8*	45	700	55	8	4.7*	1.3*	2.0*

μg/d = micrograms per day
mg/d = milligrams per day
g/d = grams per day

SAMPLE DAILY MEAL PLANS FOR FOUR DIFFERENT-SIZE TRIATHLETES

	General Recommendations	54KG (119 LBS.) FEMALE Training for a Sprint Example Guidelines for this Distance	68KG (150 LBS.) FEMALE Training for ½ IM Example Guidelines for this Distance	81KG (180 LBS.) MALE Training for IM Example Guidelines for this Distance	100KG (220 LBS.) MALE Training for Olympic Example Guidelines for this Distance
Carbohydrate	50–65% of calories 6–10g/kg	1,296 calories (50%) 324g (6g/kg)	2,176 calories (60%) 544g (8g/kg)	3,120 calories (65%) 780g (9.6g/kg)	2,820 calories (60%) 700g (7g/kg)
Protein	15–20% of calories 1.2–2.0g/kg	390 calories (15%) 97.5g (1.8g/kg)	540 calories (15%) 135g (1.9g/kg)	672 calories (14%) 168g (2.0g/kg)	720 calories (15%) 180g (1.8g/kg)
Fat	20–35% of calories	910 calories (35%)	900 calories (25%)	1,008 calories (21%)	1,175 calories (25%)
Water (not from food)*	3.0 L/d for males 2.2 L/d for females	9 cups throughout day + fluids during training	9 cups throughout day + fluids during training	12.5 cups throughout day + fluids during training	12.5 cups throughout day + fluids during training
Estimated Caloric Needs		2,600 calories /day	3,600 calories /day	4,800 calories /day	4,700 calories /day
		Sample Meal Plan	Sample Meal Plan	Sample Meal Plan	Sample Meal Plan
Breakfast		1 cup oatmeal with ½ cup blueberries, 1 oz. walnuts, & ½ cup fat-free milk 1 cup orange juice	¾ cup Kashi GOLEAN Crisp with ½ cup fat-free milk, 1 cup cranapple juice	Pancakes with butter and syrup, turkey bacon, 1 cup orange juice	3 egg omelet with cheese, mushrooms, red peppers, & 2 tsp olive oil, 2 pieces whole-wheat^ toast with butter

Breakfast Totals	530 calories, 71.5g carbohydrate 16g pro, 20g fat	365 calories, 76g carbohydrate 13g pro 3.5g fat	883 calories, 118.5g carbohydrate 20.5g pro, 35.5g fat	644 calories, 43g carbohydrate 29g pro, 35g fat
Mid-Morning Snack	Fruit smoothie (1 cup plain yogurt, ½ banana, strawberries, 1 Tbsp flaxseed oil, & 2 cups water)	2 pieces of whole-wheat toast with jelly, 2 hard-boiled eggs	1 cup Kellogg's Raisin Bran cereal with ½ cup skim milk	Whole-wheat bagel with peanut butter
Snack Totals	447 calories, 55g carbohydrate 16g pro, 16.5g fat	480 calories, 71g carbohydrate 20g pro, 13g fat	235 calories, 52.5g carbohydrate 9g pro, 1g fat	383 calories, 60g carbohydrate 14.5g pro, 10g fat
Lunch	Turkey sandwich with tomato, lettuce, and cheese on whole-wheat bread, 1 cup low-fat yogurt	Tuna-salad sandwich with mayo, lettuce, and tomato on whole-wheat bread, 1 apple, ½ cup raw carrots	1 cup pesto pasta with 4 oz. chicken (made with olive oil), vegetables and low-fat Ranch dip, 2 pieces of garlic bread	Chicken burrito from Chipotle (flour tortilla, black beans, chicken, salsa, cheese, & guacamole)
Lunch Totals	519 calories, 74g carbohydrate 17g pro, 12g fat	590 calories, 70g carbohydrate 29g pro, 9.5g fat	915 calories, 91g carbohydrate 44.5g pro, 42g fat	790 calories, 80g carbohydrate 57g pro, 25g fat
Mid-Afternoon Snack	1 Luna Bar	1 string cheese, 1 banana, & 1 oz. (24) almonds	½ cup low-fat cottage cheese with 1 cup mango	1 Clif Bar, 1 large orange
Snack Totals	180 calories, 25g carbohydrate 9g pro, 6g fat	353 calories, 34g carbohydrate 14g pro, 19g fat	197 calories, 24g carbohydrate 15g pro, 1g fat	326 calories, 66g carbohydrate 12g pro, 4.5g fat

163

SAMPLE DAILY MEAL PLANS FOR FOUR DIFFERENT-SIZE TRIATHLETES *(cont.)*

	54KG (119 LBS.) FEMALE Training for a Sprint	68KG (150 LBS.) FEMALE Training for 1/2 IM	81KG (180 LBS.) MALE Training for IM	100KG (220 LBS.) MALE Training for Olympic
	Sample Meal Plan	Sample Meal Plan	Sample Meal Plan	Sample Meal Plan
Dinner	Grilled lean-cut steak (3.5 oz.), 1/2 cup mashed potatoes, 1 cup cooked carrots & broccoli, 1 cup milk, 1/2 cup frozen yogurt	1 grilled chicken breast (4 oz.), large sweet potato with 1 oz. brown sugar & butter, salad with 2 Tbsp dressing, 2 dinner rolls with butter, 3 cookies	3 tacos (whole-wheat soft shells^ with ground turkey, cheese, lettuce, tomato, and guaca-mole), taco rice with black beans and corn, 1 cup tortilla chips and 1/4 cup salsa	Salmon fillet (4 oz.), 1.5 cups brown rice^, 1 cup mixed veggies with 2 tsp olive oil, 1 cup low-fat milk, 1 slice garlic parme-san bakery bread with butter, 1 brownie
Dinner Totals	630 calories, 63g carbohydrate 44g pro, 23g fat	1,100 calories, 117g carbohydrate 35g pro, 54.5g fat	1,274 calories, 175g carbohydrate 69.5g pro, 24.5g fat	1,276 calories, 167g carbohydrate 53.5g pro, 44g fat
Evening Snack	1 cup tortilla chips & 1/4 cup guacamole	1/2 cup low-fat cot-tage cheese with 1 cup blackberries and 1 cup raspberries	1 Clif Bar, 1 cup orange juice	1/4 muskmelon, 1/4 honeydew melon, 2 servings pretzels, 1/2 cup ice cream
Snack Totals	229 calories, 23.5g carbohydrate 3g pro, 14.5g fat	216 calories, 35g carbohydrate 17g pro, 1.5g fat	352 calories, 70g carbohydrate 12g pro, 4.5g fat	696 calories, 135g carbohydrate 16g pro, 12g fat

Daily Meal Totals	2,535 calories, 288.5g carbohydrate, 105g pro, 92g fat	3,004 calories, 403g carbohydrate, 128g pro, 101g fat	3,856 calories, 531g carbohydrate, 170.5g pro, 108.5g fat	4,115 calories, 551g carbohydrate, 182g pro, 130.5g fat
Training Food	100 calories (25g carbohydrate) for 1h workout	560 calories (140g carbohydrate) for 2h workout	980 calories (245g carbohydrate) for 3.5h workout	600 calories (150g carbohydrate) for 2.5h workout
Daily Totals	2,635 calories, 313.5g carbohydrate, 105g pro, 92g fat	3,564 calories, 543g carbohydrate, 128g pro, 101g fat	4,836 calories, 776g carbohydrate, 170.5g pro, 108.5g fat	4,715 calories, 701g carbohydrate, 182g pro, 130.5g fat

* Does not reflect water or other fluid intake during training.
^ Can substitute white to reduce fiber if it is the day before a race.

These daily meal plans do not include a specific nutrition plan for training. That information can be found in different tables in the appendix.

PRE-RACE AND PRE-TRAINING NUTRITION PLANS

Recommendations

	54KG (119 LBS.) FEMALE Training for a Sprint Race	68KG (150 LBS.) FEMALE Training for 1/2 IM Race	81KG (180 LBS.) MALE Training for IM Race	100KG (220 LBS.) MALE Training for Olympic Race
	Recommendations	**Recommendations**	**Recommendations**	**Recommendations**
Carbohydrate	1.5–2.0g/kg	2.0–3.0g/kg	2.0–3.5g/kg	1.5–2g/kg
Protein	6–20g	6–20g	6–20g	6–20g
Fat	Small amounts	Small amounts	Small amounts	Small amounts
Water (not from food)*	1–2 cups 3–4h prior 1 cup 2h prior 1 cup 30min prior	1–2 cups 3–4h prior 1 cup 2h prior 1 cup 30min prior	1–2 cups 3–4h prior 1 cup 2h prior 1 cup 30min prior	1–2 cups 3–4h prior 1 cup 2h prior 1 cup 30min prior

Sample pre-race meal for a 54kg (119-lb.) female triathlete completing a Sprint triathlon or training session of similar time

5:00 a.m (3 hours before start of race)

FOOD ITEM	SIZE	TOTAL CALORIES	CARBOHYDRATE (g)	PROTEIN (g)	FAT (g)
Plain bagel	110g	283	56g	11g	2g
Peanut butter	1 Tbsp	100	3.5g	3.5g	8g
Gatorade	240mL (1 cup)	50	14g	0g	0g
Banana	1 medium	105	27g	1g	0g
Totals		538 calories	100.5g	15.5g	10g

This meal comes out to 1.86 grams of carbohydrate per kilogram of body weight, which fits nicely into the recommended amount. She also gets a good amount of protein (fits in the 6- to 20-gram recommendation) and a small amount of fat. Additionally, she gets some electrolytes in her fluid.

Sample pre-race meal for a 68kg (150-lb.) female triathlete completing a half Ironman triathlon or training session of similar time

4:30 a.m. (2.5 hours before start of race)

FOOD ITEM	SIZE	TOTAL CALORIES	CARBOHYDRATE (g)	PROTEIN (g)	FAT (g)
Cheerios	2 cups	200	40g	6g	4g
Milk (skim)	1 cup	80	12g	8g	0g
White toast	1 slice	130	26g	4g	2g
Strawberry jam	2 Tbsp	100	26g	0g	0g
Orange juice	240mL (1 cup)	112	26g	2g	0.5g
Coffee	1 cup	0	0g	0g	0g
Totals		622 calories	143g	20g	6.5g

This meal comes out to 2.1 grams of carbohydrate per kilogram of body weight, which fits nicely into the recommended amount. She also gets a good amount of protein (fits in the 6- to 20-gram recommendation) and a small amount of fat. Since she drinks a cup of coffee, she will drink an additional cup of water before her race.

Sample pre-race meal for an 81kg (180-lb.) male triathlete completing an Ironman triathlon or a very long training session

4:30 a.m. (2.5 hours before start of race)

FOOD ITEM	SIZE	TOTAL CALORIES	CARBOHYDRATE (g)	PROTEIN (g)	FAT (g)
Boost Original*	2 bottles (~2 cups)	480	82g	20g	8g
Orange juice	240mL (1 cup)	112	26g	2g	0.5g
PowerBar Fruit Smoothie Energy bar	1 bar	220	43g	6g	3.5g
Gatorade	2 cups	100	28g	0g	0g
Totals		912 calories	179g	28g	2g

This meal comes out to 2.2 grams of carbohydrate per kilogram of body weight, which is within the lower end of the recommended amount (2.0 to 3.5 grams per kg). This meal is designed for someone who has pre-race jitters and does not have much of an appetite. If this is the case, liquid calories are a good option. Since there are quite a few liquids in this pre-race meal, the Gatorade would be consumed about two hours before the start of the race (an hour after the rest of the meal). He gets slightly more than the 6- to 20-gram recommendation for protein, but the extra grams of protein should not be detrimental (in fact, it may help since he's in for a really long day). Finally, the fat intake is relatively low and should be tolerated well, since it will be consumed three hours before the race.

* He can replace Boost with an Ensure Nutrition Shake if desired. It has the same amount of carbohydrates, and a similar total of calories, protein, and fat.

Sample pre-race meal for a 100kg (220-lb.) male triathlete completing an Olympic distance triathlon or a training session of similar time

5:00 a.m. (3.5 hours before start of race)

FOOD ITEM	SIZE	TOTAL CALORIES	CARBOHYDRATE (g)	PROTEIN (g)	FAT (g)
Eggo waffles (blueberry)	3 waffles	285	44g	6g	9g
Jam	2 Tbsp	104	26g	0g	0g
Plain English muffin	1 muffin	140	27g	5g	1g
Strawberry jam	1 Tbsp	52	13g	0g	0g
Orange juice	360mL (1.5 cup)	160	39g	4g	0g
Coffee	1 cup	0	0g	0g	0g
Totals		749 calories	149g	15g	10g

This meal comes out to 1.49 grams of carbohydrate per kilogram of body weight, which is very close to the recommended range (1.5 to 2.0 grams per kilogram of body weight). He also gets a good amount of protein (which fits in the 6- to 20-gram recommendation) and a small amount of fat. Since he drinks a cup of coffee, he will drink an additional cup of water before his race.

Other Sample Pre-Race Meals

5:00 a.m. (3.5 hours before start of race)

FOOD ITEM	SIZE	TOTAL CALORIES	CARBOHYDRATE (g)	PROTEIN (g)	FAT (g)
Quaker Instant Oatmeal, Maple and Brown Sugar	1 package	160	32g	4g	2.5g
Quaker Oats	½ cup	150	27g	5g	3g
Orange	1 large	86	22g	2g	0g
Kellogg's Pop-Tart (Frosted Brown Sugar Cinnamon)	1 pastry	210	34g	2g	7g
Luna bar	1 bar	180	27g	8g	5g
Quaker Natural Granola cereal	⅔ cup	210	44g	5g	3g
Pancakes, plain	1 pancake	86	11g	3g	4g
PB&J sandwich:					
Brownberry Oatnut bread	2 slices	240	44g	8g	5g
Strawberry jam	2 Tbsp	52	13g	0g	0g
Peanut butter	1 Tbsp	100	3.5g	3.5g	8g
Totals		392 calories	60.5g	11.5g	13g

Some of these items may be slightly higher in simple sugars, fat, or fiber, but if you don't like any of the choices from the example meals above, try a combination of foods from this list and the sample meal plans previously mentioned. Additionally, there are alternate brands that can be used as substitutes for many of those chosen here. For example, there are a number of cold cereals, bars, and breads that could easily be substituted; much of it simply depends on personal preference. Just make sure you read the labels so you know you're not getting all sugar or huge amounts of fat and fiber from the products you choose.

TRAINING AND RACING NUTRITION PLANS

Recommendations

	54KG (119 LBS.) FEMALE Training for a Sprint Race	68KG (150 LBS.) FEMALE Training for 1/2 IM Race	81KG (180 LBS.) MALE Training for IM Race	100KG (220 LBS.) MALE Training for Olympic Race
	Recommendations	Recommendations	Recommendations	Recommendations
Carbohydrate	60–70g per hour*	60–70g per hour^	60–70g per hour^	60–70g per hour^
Protein	Small amounts okay	Small amounts okay	Small amounts okay	Small amounts okay
Fat	None, or small amounts	None, or small amounts	None, or small amounts	None, or small amounts
Water (not from food)*	1 cup every 10–20 minutes	1 cup every 10–20 minutes	1 cup every 10–20 minutes	1 cup every 10–20 minutes

* Smaller amounts needed if exercising for less than ninety minutes.
^ Up to 90 grams of carbohydrate per hour is ideal, if tolerable.

Sample during-race nutrition plan for a 54kg (119-lb.) female triathlete completing a Sprint triathlon or a 60- to 90-minute training session

Expected duration: 75 minutes (1:15.00)

FOOD ITEM	RACE TIME	SIZE	TOTAL CALORIES	CARBOHYDRATE (g)	PROTEIN (g)	FAT (g)
Hammer Gel	30min	1 packet	90	22g	0g	0g
Gatorade sports drink	60min	240mL (1 cup)	50	14g	0g	0g
Water	20, 40, 80min	240mL (1 cup)	0	0	0	0
Totals			160 calories	36g	0g	0g

A race or training session of this length of time is a gray area for nutrition. Since it is less than ninety minutes, she could probably get by with water only. However, since it is over one hour in length, the carbs and calories will help ensure she finishes strong. Since the duration is short, she does not need to get 60 grams of carbohydrate per hour; the 36 grams from this sample plan is sufficient. This plan also meets her fluid needs.

171

Sample during-race nutrition plan for a 68kg (150-lb.) female triathlete completing a half Ironman triathlon or a five-hour training session

Expected duration: Five and a half hours (5:30.00)

FOOD ITEM	RACE TIME	SIZE	TOTAL CALORIES	CARBOHYDRATE (g)	PROTEIN (g)	FAT (g)
PowerBar Gel	35min	1 packet	110	27g	0g	0g
PowerBar Energy Blasts	60min	4 pieces	84	20g	1g	0g
PowerBar Fruit Smoothie Energy bar	90min	½ bar	110	21.5g	3g	2g
PowerBar Gel	120min (2h)	1 packet	110	27g	0g	0g
PowerBar Fruit Smoothie Energy bar	150min	½ bar	110	21.5g	3g	2g
PowerBar Gel	180min (3h)	1 packet	110	27g	0g	0g
PowerBar Gel	210min	1 packet	110	27g	0g	0g
PowerBar Gel	240min (4h)	1 packet	110	27g	0g	0g
PowerBar Gel	270min	1 packet	110	27g	0g	0g
PowerBar Gel	300min (5h)	1 packet	110	27g	0g	0g
Gatorade	Every 30min starting at min 45	10 cups	500	140g	0g	0g
Water	Every 20min from min 30 to min 210; then every 30min to end	13 cups	0	0	0	0
Totals			1,574 calories	392g	7g	4g

The liquid calories (Gatorade in this instance) should be consumed about halfway between each scheduled time for food consumption. For example, if you eat a gel at minutes 30 and 60, then the 1 cup of Gatorade should be at minute

45. The water intake is 1 cup every twenty minutes during the bike (from minute 30 to minute 210), and then every thirty minutes on the run (minute 210 to the end). The water intake is set up this way because it is easier to digest and absorb fluids on the bike compared to on the run. There are 23 cups of total fluid, which comes out to an average of 4.2 cups per hour. This amount should be tolerated well and also meets fluid requirements (3 to 6 cups per hour).

This nutrition plan comes out to 286 calories per hour, 71 grams of carbohydrate per hour, and very little fat or protein. This is at the upper end of the recommended intake, but if she practices with this plan, she should be able to handle it.

Sample during-race nutrition plan for an 81kg (180-lb.) male triathlete completing an Ironman distance triathlon or a very long training session

Expected Duration: Eleven Hours (11:00.00)

FOOD ITEM	RACE TIME	SIZE	TOTAL CALORIES	CARBOHYDRATE (g)	PROTEIN (g)	FAT (g)
Clif Shot Energy Gel	65min (1h)	1 packet	100	24g	0g	0g
Honey Stinger Energy Bar	90min	1 bar	180	28g	10g	3g
Clif Shot Energy Gel	120min (2h)	1 packet	100	24g	0g	0g
Clif Shot Bloks	150min	1/2 bar	100	24g	0g	0g
Jelly Belly Sport Beans	180min (3h)	1 packet	100	25g	0g	0g
Clif Shot Bloks	210min	3 pieces	100	24g	0g	0g
Cheetos Cheddar Cheese Crackers	240min (4h)	1/2 packet	105	22g	0g	6.5g
Beef Jerky		1 oz.	80	3	15	0.5
Clif Shot Bloks	270min	3 pieces	100	24g	0g	0g
Clif Shot Bloks	300min (5h)	1 packet	100	24g	0g	0g
Cheetos Cheddar Cheese Crackers	330min	1/2 packet	105	22g	0g	6.5g

173

FOOD ITEM	RACE TIME	SIZE	TOTAL CALORIES	CARBOHYDRATE (g)	PROTEIN (g)	FAT (g)
Clif Shot Bloks	360min (6h)	1 packet	100	24g	0g	0g
Honey Stinger Energy Gel	390min	1 packet	120	29g	0g	0g
Clif Shot Energy Gel	420min (7h)	1 packet	100	24g	0g	0g
Clif Shot Energy Gel	450min	1 packet	100	24g	0g	0g
Chicken Broth		½ cup	19	0.5	2.5	0.5
Honey Stinger Energy Gel	480min (8h)	1 packet	120	29g	0g	0g
Clif Shot Energy Gel	510min	1 packet	100	24g	0g	0g
Clif Shot Energy Gel	540min (9h)	1 packet	100	24g	0g	0g
Cola (flat)		½ cup	50	13.5	0	0
Honey Stinger Energy Gel	570min	1 packet	120	29g	0g	0g
Clif Shot Energy Gel	600min (10h)	1 packet	100	24g	0g	0g
Clif Shot Energy Gel	630min	1 packet	100	24g	0g	0g
PowerBar Ironman Perform Sports Drink	2 cups per hour starting at 1h	20 cups	1,400	340g	0g	0g
Water	2 cups per hour from hours 1–6; 1.5 cups per hour from hours 6–11	17.5 cups	0	0	0	0
Totals			3,699 calories	853g	27.5g	16.5g

This IM triathlete begins consuming calories as soon as he is finished with the swim (in this example, it is at sixty-five minutes). There are more solid foods on the bike and then mostly gels and liquids on the run. This is because it is generally easier to chew food and digest and absorb more food on the bike compared to the run. Additionally, having different types of food, gels, and liquids throughout the day should help prevent flavor fatigue. The salty foods (beef jerky and chicken broth) are there to help prevent flavor fatigue. The beef jerky and crackers are around hour 4, so the triathlete is able to pick up those items in his bike special needs bag. For the run, gels and liquids are what he consumes. He also takes on a little cola to help settle his stomach. He consumes a mix of water and sports drink throughout the day. While on the bike, he drinks about 4 cups per hour. For the run, he backs off slightly and drinks about 3.5 cups per hour because it is a little harder to digest and absorb as much fluid during running versus biking.

For this nutrition plan, he is getting an average of 336 calories per hour, 77.5 grams of carbohydrate per hour, 3.5 cups of fluid per hour, a little protein, and just a small amount of fat. This is slightly higher than the 60- to 70-gram recommendation for carbohydrates, but it is actually beneficial to get up to 90 grams of carbohydrates per hour if the athlete can tolerate it.

Sample during-race nutrition for a 100kg (220-lb.) male triathlete completing an Olympic distance triathlon or a three-hour training session

Expected duration: Three hours (3:00.00)

FOOD ITEM	RACE TIME	SIZE	TOTAL CALORIES	CARBOHYDRATE (g)	PROTEIN (g)	FAT (g)
Accel Gel	30min	1 packet	90	20g	5g	0g
GU Chomps	60min (1h)	4 pieces	90	23g	0g	0g
GU Chomps	90min	4 pieces	90	23g	0g	0g
GU Chomps	120min (2h)	4 pieces	90	23g	0g	0g
Accel Gel	150min	1 packet	90	20g	5g	0g
Powerade Sports Drink	Every 30min starting at min 45	5 cups	250	70g	0g	0g
Water	Every 30min starting at min 30	5 cups	0	0	0	0
Totals			700 calories	179g	10g	0g

This triathlete begins taking on calories thirty minutes into the training session (or, if it's a race, soon after he gets on the bike). There are more liquid calories in this plan, so some of the food items are split up between two eating times. Further, there are some solid foods on the bike, but only liquids and a gel for the run (this helps to prevent flavor fatigue). The easiest things to digest and absorb will be consumed while running. Between the Powerade and water, he consumes 3 to 4 cups of fluid per hour: 3 cups in hour 1 (2 cups water, 1 cup Powerade), 4 cups in hour 2 (2 cups water, 2 cups Powerade), and 3 cups in hour 3 (1 cup water, 2 cups Powerade). This nutrition plan comes out to 233 calories per hour, 60 grams of carbohydrate per hour, has some protein, and contains no fat.

POST-RACE AND POST-TRAINING NUTRITION PLANS

Recommendations

	54KG (119 LBS.) FEMALE Sprint Distance Race	68KG (150 LBS.) FEMALE Half Ironman Race	81KG (180 LBS.) MALE Full IM Race	100KG (220 LBS.) MALE Olympic Distance Race
	Recommendations	**Recommendations**	**Recommendations**	**Recommendations**
Carbohydrate	1.2g/kg	1.2g/kg	1.2g/kg	1.2g/kg
Protein	6-20g	6-20g	6-20g	6-20g
Fat	Small amounts	Small amounts	Small amounts	Small amounts
Water	2-3 cups for each pound of body weight lost	2-3 cups for each pound of body weight lost	2-3 cups for each pound of body weight lost	2-3 cups for each pound of body weight lost

Sample post-race meal for a 54kg (119-lb.) female triathlete completing a Sprint triathlon or a training session of similar time

15 to 30 minutes post-race

FOOD ITEM	SIZE	TOTAL CALORIES	CARBOHYDRATE (g)	PROTEIN (g)	FAT (g)
Athletes HoneyMilk	1 bottle (340mL)	340	26g	26g	3.5g
Banana	1 medium	105	27g	1g	0g
Gatorade	1 cup (240mL)	50	14g	0g	0g
Water	2 cups	0	0	0	0
Totals		495 calories	67g	27g	3.5g

This athlete needs to have 65 grams of carbohydrate to meet the recommendation of 1.2 grams per kilogram of body weight, so this meal meets her initial needs. It is also heavy on the liquid calories, which should make it easier to consume right after an intense race. The protein is slightly higher than the 6- to 20-gram recommendation, but that will not do any harm to her recovery. Dietary fat is low, which will help with speedy digestion and absorption of carbohydrates and proteins. She also gets electrolytes and plenty of water to replenish those lost during racing.

Sample post-race meal for a 68kg (150-lb.) female triathlete completing a half Ironman triathlon or a training session of similar time

15 to 30 minutes post-race

FOOD ITEM	SIZE	TOTAL CALORIES	CARBOHYDRATE (g)	PROTEIN (g)	FAT (g)
Carnation Breakfast Essentials Drink (Classic French Vanilla)	1 bottle (325mL)	250	34g	14g	5g
Pretzels	2 oz. (17 pretzels)	110	23g	2g	1g
Kellogg's Pop-Tart (Frosted Brown Sugar Cinnamon)	1 pastry	210	34g	2g	7g
Water	2 cups	0	0	0	0
Totals		570 calories	91g	18g	13g

This triathlete needs to have 82 grams of carbohydrate to meet the recommendation of 1.2 grams per kilogram of body weight, so this meal meets her initial needs. It has a combination of both liquid calories and solid foods that are high in sugar. The protein meets the recommended amount of 6 to 20 grams, and the dietary fat intake should not interfere greatly with the digestion and absorption of the other nutrients. Remember that this carbohydrate and protein recommendation should be consumed every hour for about two to three hours post-race.

Sample post-race meal for an 81kg (180-lb.) male triathlete completing an Ironman triathlon or a very long training session

15 to 30 minutes post-race

FOOD ITEM	SIZE	TOTAL CALORIES	CARBOHYDRATE (g)	PROTEIN (g)	FAT (g)
Low-fat chocolate milk	2 cups (480mL)	316	52g	16g	5g
Soft pretzel	1 small	210	43g	5g	2g
Gatorade	1 cup	50	14g	0g	0g
Totals		576 calories	109g	21g	7g

This triathlete needs to have 97 grams of carbohydrate to meet the recommendation of 1.2 grams per kilogram of body weight, so this meal meets his initial needs. It has a combination of both liquid calories and solid foods, with plenty of electrolytes (especially sodium) in the Gatorade and pretzel. The protein meets the recommended amount of 6 to 20 grams, and the dietary fat intake is low, which will not delay the digestion and absorption of carbohydrates and proteins. Remember that this carbohydrate and protein recommendation should be consumed every hour for about three to four hours post-race.

Sample post-race meal for a 100kg (220-lb.) male triathlete completing an Olympic distance triathlon or a training session of similar time

15 to 30 minutes post-race

FOOD ITEM	SIZE	TOTAL CALORIES	CARBOHYDRATE (g)	PROTEIN (g)	FAT (g)
Carnation Breakfast Essentials Drink (Rich Chocolate Milk)	1 bottle (325mL)	260	41g	14g	5g
Bagel, blueberry	1 bagel	250	54g	9g	1.5g
Chocolate chip cookies	2 small cookies (12g each)	114	16g	2g	6g
Gatorade	240mL (1 cup)	50	14g	0g	0g
Water	3 cups	0	0	0	0
Totals		674 calories	125g	25g	12.5g

This triathlete needs to have 120 grams of carbohydrate to meet the recommendation of 1.2 grams per kilogram of body weight, so this meal meets his initial recovery needs. It has a combination of both liquid calories and solid food, so it's easy to eat right after a fairly intense race. The protein is slightly higher than the 6- to 20-gram recommendation, but that will not do any harm to his recovery. Dietary fat is fairly low with this meal, so it shouldn't delay digestion and absorption of carbohydrates and proteins. He also gets electrolytes and plenty of water to replenish those lost during the race.

There are several other foods or combinations of foods and liquids that would work for post-race meals. Calculate your carbohydrate needs and then make sure the meal meets those carbohydrate needs, has 6 to 20 grams of protein, and has a small amount of fat. Try to focus on high-glycemic-index (high-sugar) foods for this first meal.

COMMON SALT AND ELECTROLYTE TABLET PRODUCTS

BRAND NAME	SODIUM	POTASSIUM	CHLORIDE	OTHER
BASE Electrolyte Salt	290mg	2.6mg	442mg	Ca^{2+} 3mg, Mg^{2+} 12mg
BioSalt Tabs (ProHealth)	180mg	15mg		
CamelBak Elixir	340mg	125mg		
Electrolyte Stamina (Trace Minerals Research)	270mg	590mg	1370mg	Ca^{2+} 400mg, Mg^{2+} 290mg
Elete Tablytes	150mg	95mg	350mg	Ca^{2+} 40mg, Mg^{2+} 30mg
Essential electrolytes (Nutribiotics)	53mg	75mg	79mg	Ca^{2+} 50mg, Mg^{2+} 25mg
First Aid Only Electrolyte Tablets		40mg		CaPhosphate 18mg, Mg^{2+} 9mg
GU Brew Electrolyte Tablets	320mg	55mg		
Hammer Nutrition Endurolytes	40mg	25mg	60mg	Ca^{2+} 50mg, Mg^{2+} 25mg
HyLytes	50mg	25mg		Ca^{2+} 25mg, Mg^{2+} 25mg
Lava Salts (Squeezy)	225mg	30mg		
Medi-Lyte		40mg		CaPhosphate 18mg, MgC 9mg
Motor Tabs	250mg	75mg		
Nathan Catalyst	135mg	60mg		
NUUN	175mg	50mg		Ca^{2+} 12.5mg, Mg^{2+} 12.5mg
Peltier Ultra	68mg	94mg	74mg	Mg^{2+} 10mg
Salt Stick Caps	215mg	63mg		Ca^{2+} 22mg, Mg^{2+} 11mg

BRAND NAME	SODIUM	POTASSIUM	CHLORIDE	OTHER
Shotz	215mg	21mg		Ca^{2+} 6.25mg, Mg^{2+} 10mg
Succeed S Caps	341mg	21mg		
Swift Electrolyte Tablets	220mg	15mg		Ca^{2+}C 18mg
Thermolyte MetaSalt	330mg	85.2mg		Ca^{2+} 25.2mg
Thermotabs	180mg	15mg	287mg	
ZYM	250mg	50mg		Ca^{2+} 30mg, Mg^{2+} 50mg

COMMON RECOVERY PRODUCTS

PRODUCT	SERVING SIZE	CALORIES	CARBOHYDRATES (g)	PROTEIN (g)	FAT (g)	SODIUM (mg)
Athletes HoneyMilk	1 bottle (340mL)	240	26g	26g	3.5g	120mg
Boost Plus	1 bottle (237ml)	360	45g	14g	14g	200mg
Carnation Breakfast Essentials Drink (Classic French Vanilla)	1 bottle (325mL)	250	34g	14g	5g	180mg
Carnation Breakfast Essentials Drink (Rich Chocolate Milk)	1 bottle (325mL)	260	41g	14g	5g	230mg
Champion Nutrition Metabolol II (rich chocolate)	2 scoops (66g)	260	40g	18g	3	200mg
Endurox R4 Recovery Drink	2 rounded scoops (74g)	270	52g	13g	1.5g	190mg
Ensure (vanilla)	1 bottle (8 oz.)	250	40g	9g	6g	200mg
First Endurance Ultragen	2 scoops (12 oz.)	320	60g	20g	0g	350mg
Gatorade Recover (G Series)	1 bottle (8 oz.)	60	7g	8g	0g	120mg
Gatorade Recover (G Series Pro)	1 bottle (8 oz.)	110	20g	8g	0g	105mg
GU Recovery Brew	3 scoops (60g)	250	52g	8g	0g	160mg
Hammer Nutrition Recoverite	2 scoops (49g)	170	31g	10g	0g	40mg
Low-Fat Chocolate Milk (Nesquik)	1 bottle (8 oz.)	170	29g	8g	2.5g	160mg
Shaklee Physique	4 scoops (8 oz.)	210	38g	14g	0g	80mg
Ultra Fuel (Twin Labs)	2 scoops (16 oz.)	400	100g	0g	0g	60mg

COMMON SPORTS PERFORMANCE PRODUCTS

PRODUCT GELS	SERVING SIZE/ SERVINGS PER CONTAINER	CALORIES	CARBOHYDRATE (g)	PROTEIN (g)	TOTAL FAT (g)	SODIUM (mg)	CHLORIDE (mg)	POTASSIUM (mg)	CAFFEINE (mg)
2nd Surge	1 pk (29g) /1	90	18g	3g	0g	115mg		15mg	100mg
Accel Gel	1 pk (37g) /1	100	20g	5g	0g	115mg		20mg	0–40mg
Carb BOOM!	1 pk (41g) /1	110	27g	0g	0g	50mg		50mg	0–50mg
Clif Shot Energy Gel	1 pk (34g) /1	100	24g	0g	0g	60mg		80mg	0–100mg
Clif Shot Turbo Energy Gel	1 pk (34g) /1	110	22g	0g	1.5g	60mg		85mg	100mg
GU Energy Gel	1 pk (32g) /1	100	25g	0g	0g	50mg		40mg	
GU Roctane Ultra Endurance	1 pk (32g) /1	100	25g		2g	125mg		55mg	35mg
Hammer Nutrition Gel	1.7 Tbsp (32.9g) /1	90	21g			25mg		25mg	0–50mg
Honey Stinger Energy Gel	1 pk (37g) /1	120	29g	0g	0g	50mg		85mg	
PowerBar Gel	1 pk (41g) /1	110	27g	0g	0g	200mg		20mg	0–50mg
Lava Gel (Squeezy)	1 pk (34g) /1	100	25g	Cg	0g	120mg	75mg	30mg	

185

COMMON SPORTS PERFORMANCE PRODUCTS *(cont.)*

PRODUCT SPORTS BARS	SERVING SIZE/ SERVINGS PER CONTAINER	CALORIES	CARBOHYDRATE (g)	PROTEIN (g)	TOTAL FAT (g)	SODIUM (mg)	CHLORIDE (mg)	POTASSIUM (mg)	CAFFEINE (mg)
Clif Bar	1 bar (68g)/1	240	44g	10g	4.5g	150mg		210mg	
Hammer Nutrition Bar	1 bar (50g)/1	220	26g	10g	9g	18mg			
Honey Stinger Energy Bar	1 bar (50g)/1	180	28g	10g	3g	160mg		130mg	
Kashi Go Lean	1 bar (55g)/1	190	31g	12g	4.5g	120mg		130mg	
Larabar	1 bar (45g)/1	220	28g	4g	11g	55mg		320mg	
Luna Bar	1 bar (48g)/1	180	27g	8g	5g	115mg		105mg	
Met-RX Protein Plus	1 bar (85g)/1	320	33g	32g	10g	290mg		200mg	
Odwalla Protein Bar	1 bar (56g)/1	210	36g	5g	6g	210mg		210mg	
PowerBar Performance Energy Bars	1 bar (60g)/1	240	45g	8g	3.5g	200mg		105mg	
Zone Perfect	1 bar (50g)/1	210	24g	14g	7g	270mg		130mg	

OTHER PRODUCTS	SERVING SIZE/ SERVINGS PER CONTAINER	CALORIES	CARBOHYDRATE (g)	PROTEIN (gr)	TOTAL FAT (g)	SODIUM (mg)	CHLORIDE (mg)	POTASSIUM (mg)	CAFFEINE (mg)
Carb BOOM! Energy chews	6 pieces (30g)/1	90	23g	0g	0g	55mg		40mg	
Clif Shot Bloks	3 pieces (30g)/2	100	24g	0g	0g	70mg		20mg	
Clif Shot Roks	10 pieces (70g)/1	270	37g	20g	4.5g	330mg		85mg	
GU Chomps	4 pieces (30g)/2	90	23g	0g	0g	50mg		40mg	
Hammer Nutrition Perpetuem Solids	3 tablets (25.5)	100	20g	3g	0.9g	81mg		28mg	10mg
Honey Stinger Organic Energy Chews	10 pieces (50g)	160	39g	1g	0g	80mg		40mg	
Jelly Belly Sport Beans	1 pk (28g)/1	100	25g	0g	0g	80mg		40mg	
PowerBar Energy Bites	4 pieces(42g)/2	150	26g	5g	3g	125mg		0mg	
PowerBar Energy Blasts	9 pieces (60g)/1	190	45g	3g	0g	60mg		0mg	
Sharkies Organic Energy Fruit Chews	1 pk (45g)/1	140	36g	0g	0g	110mg		30mg	

Some products contain caffeine, depending on which flavor is chosen. In addition, slightly different nutritional information exists for different flavors of the same product, so read the labels carefully.

COMMON SPORTS BEVERAGES

PRODUCT	CARBOHYDRATE (g)	TYPE OF CARBOHYDRATE	SODIUM (mg)	POTASSIUM (mg)	VITAMINS AND MINERALS	OTHER INGREDIENTS
Accelerade	14	Sucrose, fructose, trehalose	127	43	67% of DV for vitamins C and E	3.3g protein
All Sport Body Quencher	16	High-fructose corn syrup	55	60	40% of DV for vitamin C	None
Carbo-Pro	19	Glucose polymers	0	0	None	None
Extran Thirstquencher	7	Fructose, maltodextrin	96	28	None	None
Gatorade (G Series Pro) 02 Performance (Endurance)	14	Sucrose, fructose	200	90	Small amounts of calcium and magnesium added	None
Gatorade Thirst Quencher	14	Sucrose, dextrose	110	30	None	None
Hammer Nutrition Heed	20	Maltodextrin, zylitol, stevia	30	12	Added magnesium, vitamin B6, manganese, and chromium	None
High 5 Isotonic	19	Maltodextrin, fructose	200	58	None	None
PowerBar Ironman Perform	17	Maltodextrin, dextrose, fructose	190	10	Added magnesium	None
Powerade	19	High-fructose corn syrup, maltodextrin	55	30	10% vitamin B6, B12, and niacin	None
Shaklee Performance	25	Maltodextrin, fructose, glucose	130	50	Added calcium, magnesium, and phosphorus	None

Glossary

Carbohydrate and glycogen loading: Process of storing extra amounts of carbohydrate in the body.

Electrolytes: A substance that contains free ions. In the body, these are important for nerve impulse transmission, fluid balance, muscle contraction, and molecule movement into and out of cells. The primary electrolytes of interest for athletes include sodium, chloride, and potassium.

Energy (calorie) content of food:
> There are 4 calories per gram of protein.
> There are 4 calories per gram of carbohydrate.
> There are 7 calories per gram of alcohol.
> There are 9 calories per gram of fat.

Enzyme: Protein that helps a reaction occur in the body.

Ergogenic Aids: Something external (outside of the body) that can enhance performance.

GI (gastrointestinal) distress: Problems in the digestive tract, including nausea, vomiting, bloating, cramping, gas, and diarrhea.

Glycogen: The storage form of carbohydrate in your body. You can store carbohydrates in your liver and muscle.

Macronutrient: A nutrient (carbohydrate, fat, or protein) that gives your body a large amount of energy and something your body needs in large amounts in order to function properly.

Metabolism: Chemical reactions that occur in the body to keep you alive and to keep your body systems functioning.

Micronutrient: A nutrient (vitamins, minerals) that does not provide any energy but that your body still needs in small amounts in order to function properly.

Recommended Intakes:
> The DRIs (dietary reference intakes) is an umbrella term used to describe a number of different terms for recommended intakes of nutrients. These other terms include the RDA, and the AI.

> The RDA (recommended dietary allowance) is the amount of a nutrient that will meet the needs of 98 percent of healthy individuals.

> The AI (adequate intake) is the amount of a nutrient that is commonly eaten in a healthy population of people who are free from disease. The AI is basically set when there is not enough science/research to determine what an RDA should be for a given nutrient. So, the AI is probably an adequate amount of that nutrient for your body to function properly.

Red Zone: A high intensity of exercise that cannot be sustained for long periods of time. This is usually above an athlete's lactate or ventilatory threshold, and as such, heart rate and breathing rate are quite high.

Index

About the Author

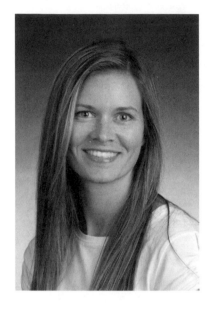

JAMIE COOPER, PHD, received her bachelor's and master's degrees in exercise physiology from Michigan State University and her PhD in nutritional sciences from the University of Wisconsin-Madison. She is currently an assistant professor at Texas Tech University, where she teaches undergraduate and graduate courses in Sports Nutrition, Issues in Sports Nutrition, and Sports Supplements and Ergogenic Aids. Jamie has also been coaching triathletes, runners, and fitness enthusiasts (both in training and nutrition) for several years. She completed her first marathon at the age of eighteen and started competing in triathlons in 2005. She has completed a number of marathons, including the Boston Marathon, as well as a number of triathlons. She enjoys competing in all distance triathlons, ranging from sprints to Ironman distance, and has done Ironman Wisconsin two times, Ironman Canada once, and Ironman Louisville once. She enjoys training with her husband, also an Ironman triathlete, and likes to put her nutrition knowledge and practice to the test in order to help others reach their athletic goals.